Heaven Sent

Soul Lessons from the Afterlife

Claire Broad

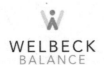

WELBECK
BALANCE

Published in 2023 by Welbeck Balance
An imprint of Welbeck Non-Fiction Limited
Part of Welbeck Publishing Group
Offices in: London – 20 Mortimer Street, London W1T 3JW &
Sydney – Level 17, 207 Kent St, Sydney NSW 2000 Australia
www.welbeckpublishing.com

A CIP catalogue record for this book is available from the British Library.

ISBN
978-1-80129-271-9

Typeset by Lapiz Digital Services
Printed in Great Britain by CPI Group (UK) Ltd, Croydon CRO 4YY

10 9 8 7 6 5 4 3 2 1

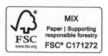

MIX
Paper | Supporting
responsible forestry
FSC® C171272

Note/Disclaimer

Dedicated to the adventures of the
twenty-two with two little ducks.

Contents

Setting the Intention

I feel the need to start this introduction by highlighting that this book is not intended to be autobiographical. Although the teachings I share are written from the benefit of real-life hands-on experience, the book's message is about something so much greater than my own individual soul journey, and certainly far more encompassing. I share the true life stories of clients, students and members of the public – with permission – instead of my own personal life stories, to integrate understanding. My own experiences are then offered purely where necessary to reinforce the teaching, in an attempt to distance the medium from the message.

To help you understand how I became qualified to teach about the soul and soul connections, I believe it will be helpful to provide you with a brief history here in this introduction.

Introduction

How would you feel if I said I could offer you the most incredible journey of a lifetime? That this adventure, however, would require that you take the rough with the smooth in order to provide you with an experience that would ultimately lead you to more bliss, peace, love, empowerment, contentment, pleasure and euphoria than any holiday in paradise ever could? And what if I told you that this grandest of adventures would include a short stay on a gigantic rock that hurtles though space without a driver. Would you find that a thrilling prospect and sign up? Or would you turn away from the offer thinking it was pure madness? Well … I'm going to suggest that you are already signed up and, here you are, journeying on Earth with the rest of us souls as we experience the ride of our lives!

***

We somehow expect our loved ones to always be there, and it's often not until they die – or there is a painful parting of the ways – that many of us turn our attention to the spiritual dimension of life. This is when people find me. If a loved one has passed away, a client may look to reconnect with them through my ability in mediumship. They seek reassurance that their loved one is happy in the afterlife and knows how much they are loved. It's amazing how many of us in this world don't express our heartfelt emotions to our closest loved ones until it's too late. By coming to see me, I help clients know that their spirit loved ones are well, and that the love between them is unconditional, even after physical death. I am able to tell them of their "soul connection" – when two people meet and resonate so well together that they form an energetic soul bond that transcends death. This connection at the heart and soul, is eternal.

For other clients, if relationships with family, friends or romantic partners have become strained or even estranged before a person dies, I can help them to understand the deeper "soul lessons" learned from the challenges in these connections. For example, someone may come to me having lost a parent with whom they had a difficult relationship. This does not mean that the child stopped loving the parent, or the parent's love for the child ended. Once the parent has died, what once was an insurmountable rift may no longer seem so important. Issues that were cause for argument become water under the bridge. In these circumstances, those in the spirit world are often keen to reach out to right wrongdoing and take responsibility for their part. Spirit guides work with me, highlighting the spiritual gains despite the earthly losses. I have found such insight brings healing and peace. This greater soul perspective allows people to let go of fear, guilt and pain that they no longer need to carry.

Others come to see me because they are ready to understand more about their own soul and their spiritual life purpose. In soul guidance sessions, I work with the spirit guides to gain insight into these clients' soul journeys, as well as exploring why their soul came here in this lifetime with the significant people they have in their lives. The spirit world helps me to make sense of the type of soul connections being shared between my clients and other souls – both in this world and the next. They also help me to understand the "soul purpose" underpinning these relationships. Sometimes insights given extend back to previous lifetimes spent together, and the spirit guides will also relay insight about those lifetimes too, in order to help make greater sense of the life challenges experienced in this lifetime. Often clients are seeking greater understanding from a spiritual perspective as they try to navigate challenging soul connections in life – an intense love affair ending without warning perhaps, or a controlling friendship creating great heartache. Working with the insight I receive from spirit guides I pass on the wisdom given to help clients live and love more fearlessly, and to realize their eternal soul self.

Spirit messenger

I am one of those people – I see now with hindsight – who was born into this world with a spiritual calling to be a teacher and practitioner for the spirit world. That calling revealed itself to me from a very early age – as from the age of two (and quite possibly from birth) I have been able to sense the souls of the "dead" around me.

At age two, I regularly pointed out to my mum, the man I could see in my bedroom. Of course, she could not see anyone there and was puzzled, but I was adamant! Then, at the age of four, I "heard" my deceased grandad communicating with me, conveying a message of love to my Nan from beyond the grave.

I have written extensively about these and many other early personal experiences with the spirit world in *What The Dead Are Dying To Teach Us: Lessons Learned From The Afterlife* and in *Answers From Heaven: Incredible True Stories of Heavenly Encounters and the Afterlife*. I've also spoken on many radio shows, podcasts and to the press, to the fact throughout my life, I have had experiences that helped me to realize the reality and existence of the spirit world.

As a consequence of being able to sense the spirit world around me, I have the privilege of being guided directly by a team of highly evolved spiritual beings. This guidance began when a spirit intelligence introduced himself as "White Feather" (the meaning behind the name is spiritual symbolism because white feathers often denote the connection between the spirit world and Earth). White Feather first appeared to me as an apparition in my teenage years, and despite my reluctance to engage with him due to fear he endeavoured to prove his existence through a series of highly unusual events (also written about in *What The Dead Are Dying To Teach Us*). His presence utterly terrified me at first, as it would any teen with little understanding of spirit communication and the afterlife.

At my first ever mediumship appointment at the age of 19, White Feather communicated directly through the medium carrying out the reading, asking her to please take me under her wing so I could develop my own ability as a channel for the spirit world safely. Thus began what has turned out to be an incredible "otherworldly" union between White Feather and myself. His wisdom and guidance, always delivered with a wonderful sense of humour, has remained steady. I find it incredible that, as down to earth and as rational as I am, I can say with all seriousness that I have experienced unwavering support and pure soul love from an intelligence that is not in physical form.

I am now supported by a whole team of spirit guides and master teachers, each with their own area of responsibility in helping me accomplish my spiritual work, and all of whom have managed in their own way to prove their existence to me. Of course, I wouldn't ask anyone else to believe what I'm saying without question. I understand that what I say may seem unfathomable to some – I can only openly share and say: this is my truth and reality. You must be free to draw your own conclusions about the truth in my words and the reality of the spirit world, for yourself.

As to my credentials, I am now a professional medium, having been accredited as a Registered and Approved Medium by the Institute of Spiritualist Mediums in the UK, trained in Evidence-Based Mediumship (the practice of relaying messages from souls of the deceased to the souls of the living, containing information the medium could not know by usual means, thereby providing evidence suggestive of the survival of consciousness after death) within The Spiritualist National Union. I am also a trainer at the world-famous College of Psychic Studies in London, humbly walking with reverence in the footsteps of such historical greats as the renowned creator of Sherlock Holmes, Sir Arthur Conan Doyle; the Rev. William Stainton Moses, a phenomenal medium of his time; and chemist and physicist Sir William Crookes.

For over 25 years now, I have received instruction directly from White Feather and the wider team of spirit teachers in the spirit world that accompany me. In that time, I have been privileged to deliver thousands of messages to members of the general public during private appointments, teaching events and public demonstrations.

The missing piece of the puzzle
After the release of my previous books, a wonderful shift happened. A good number of clients began visiting or returning to my private practice, already confident that the afterlife is real. These clients came trusting that their loved ones lived on, and so

were seeking a deeper and more insightful experience from my services than I had traditionally offered in my evidence-based mediumship sessions. As a result, it became glaringly obvious to me that there had been a missing piece to the puzzle. It wasn't enough to simply gain understanding of life after death and the spirit world. As impressive as evidence of survival is, there was much more that needed to be passed on in order to help others.

Understanding the soul and soul connections became central to my teaching. In helping people attain greater understanding of their own soul, their soul journey and the unconditional love that they are, they learned to see life from a greater soul perspective. In turn, this helped them make sense of their own life circumstances in a way they hadn't considered before – empowering them and granting greater wisdom, inner peace and emotional freedom. The soul was the missing piece.

The spirit guides find their way to you

The spirit guides have guided me back to writing again to pass on to you the understanding they have taught me about the eternal soul and the giving of unconditional love, both to yourself as well as to others. In guiding your understanding about the most common soul connections you will likely experience in your own life and their purposes, the spirit guides can also educate you about the ultimate purpose for your soul, and for all souls.

This book has been written to help those who have lost loves from their life and all those keen to gain deeper spiritual wisdom and insight from the spirit world in order to understand relationships more soulfully. You can absorb more about your own soul and unconditional love; and understand the commitments of "Soul Family", "Karmic partners", "Catalysts", "Life Partners",

"Soulmates" and "Twin Flames". Who doesn't ask themselves the deeper questions such as, "What is it all about?", "Will I be loved?", "Why am I here?" and "Am I achieving my life purpose?" Your soul is calling you to this information on its path toward lasting spiritual enlightenment and remembrance of a universal love so powerful that even death holds no limitation for its reach. It's wonderful to have you here to journey with me for a while …

Glossary of Useful Terms

When we form relationships with other people, we naturally form bonds that are not just emotional ties but also energetic ties. The energy of both souls unties and the bond created forms what are known as soul connections. One of the best ways to know the reality of your own eternal soul is to see or sense another's soul reflected back at you while in soul connection. What's fascinating is that there are so many types of soul connections – each with their own distinct dynamic.

In this book I will cover the most common soul connections people experience: Soul Family and Earth Family, Karmic and Catalyst soul connections, Life Partners and Soulmates, plus Twin Flames/Twin Souls. Those in the spirit world teach that because of soul connections, souls journey together (often through many lifetimes) in order to learn from one another and grow in soul awareness, as well as in pure love. I will explain this further as we go through the book, but I thought it would be helpful for you to have a glossary of the terms I use regularly. If you come across a term that isn't clear, return here for a simple reminder of the meaning.

- Catalyst Soul Connection – An intense relationship between two people that begins with pure soul love but ends abruptly and painfully.
- Ego Death – The letting go of deep-rooted thoughts and perspectives held in your mind that have shaped your personality in the past but no longer reflect who you are as a soul.
- Earth Family – Relationships you share with biological family members with whom you do not share strong soul bonds.
- Karmic Soul Connection – A relationship that was formed in a previous lifetime and which you continue to learn and grow from in this lifetime.
- Life Partner Soul Connection – A loving romantic relationship that is stable and lasts a lifetime but which also supports freedom, independence and individual soul growth.
- Over-Soul – A collection of soul groups as well as the sum total of all souls.
- Primordial Source Energy – The energy from which everything in the universe emerges.
- Romantic Soulmate Soul Connection – A romantic relationship that is intensely loving and supportive, and in which both people involved choose to do as much together as possible because one can't live happily without the other.
- Shadow Work – Self-reflection and transformation of the negative aspects of your personality that keep you locked in fearful behaviour and away from love.
- Soul Activation – When your soul recognizes the soul energy of another person as a soul you have met in a prior lifetime and activates the soul memory, or when your soul

recognizes its exact same soul energy in another person
(as in the case of Twin Flames).

- Soul Agreement – The agreement two souls share to come
  into a physical life together and journey for a period of
  time with a particular purpose.
- Soul Awareness – Becoming mentally aware that you are a
  soul, and growing in understanding about what the soul is
  trying to achieve in life, while learning to live in alignment
  with the soul and in balance with the thinking mind.
- Soul Bond – An emotional and energetic connection
  between two people that transcends death.
- Spirit Communication – The passing on of information and
  wisdom from the spirit world to this world.
- Soul Connection – When two people meet and resonate
  so well together that they form an energetic soul bond
  that transcends death.
- Soul Family – The souls that form the closest and most
  loving relationships in your life (this can be biological
  family or friends).
- Soul Group – A collective of souls of which your soul is
  part.
- Soul Guidance – Wisdom received from the spirit
  world about your soul journey in this lifetime and
  previous lifetimes.
- Soul Heal – To heal at the deepest level of your soul, not
  just physically or mentally, but spiritually too.
- Soul Journey – The journey a soul takes throughout many
  lifetimes, and also in the spirit world, on a pathway to
  understanding the soul self.
- Soul Lessons – Lessons we learn while we experience life
  here before returning to the spirit world.

- Soul Love – Pure, unconditional, eternal love.
- Soul Memory – The information your soul stores throughout many lifetimes of experiences.
- Soul Merge – When two souls blend together perfectly in energy and, for a while, become like one soul.
- Soulmate Soul Connections – Your closest and most harmonious relationships.
- Twin Flame/Twin Soul/Mirror Soul Connections – One soul divided into two mirror counterparts or twins, which then incarnate as two separate people.

Chapter One

You Are An Eternal Soul

"Begin to see yourself as a soul with a body,
rather than a body with a soul."
Wayne Dyer

This book is about *you*. The eternal you. The soul you. This you is truly awesome. So awesome in fact that the conscious mind might not be able to easily grasp the full reality of who you really are – and maybe it never will. "Awesome" is a word overused these days, rendering the power of the word much less impactful than it would have been in the past; but when I use the word here I really do mean you are AWESOME. I am in awe of you, and when you truly realize the incredible, indestructible nature of who you really are, you'll be in awe of you too.

In this book, I will guide you towards a recognition of your eternal soul self and help you gain a greater understanding of the power of pure soul love. I hope, through doing so, you will acquire confidence that love never dies, and you will live life more soul aware.

To be soul aware is to know you are a soul who inhabited the spirit world before entering your life here. I will share with you how your soul entered into this world, coming here with great purpose and meaning. I will also highlight some of the soul lessons you came to master with those you love (or have loved) in your life. As an extension to this, I will also help you identify for yourself the many soul connections you have made and help you learn their soul purpose. By the end of your journey with me, you will have grasped a greater appreciation of how truly awesome you are as an eternal soul and gained deeper insight into your own soul journey, so that you can embrace life more fearlessly and fully because now you understand … you are heaven sent.

I will begin by helping you to comprehend the eternal nature of your own soul through this chapter, bringing insights to you from those in the spirit world who return to provide us with evidence that the soul is indestructible and love never dies. I will also help you to see from the perspective of your own soul and to appreciate that you are much more than this physical body. This will provide the foundation you need to enjoy and understand the chapters that follow regarding pure soul love and your own eternal soul connections.

The soul is real

As a spirit messenger and spiritual teacher, I have dedicated my life to educating others that they are not just a physical being, but a spiritual being too. The afterlife is real, and at your time of death your soul will release from the physical body and transition into a spiritual light body. Your soul will then journey into the realms of the afterlife to be reunited with those you love.

We don't need to wait until we die to learn the truth of this. It is possible to feel connected with the spirit world right now, and to learn from the insights brought to you from the souls who reach out to comfort, support and educate you from beyond the veil. Their loving communications teach us the soul is real, and that your soul entered into this world in order to have all manner of experiences, helping you evolve into greater levels of soul awareness.

The doorway to eternity

I'm a regular person despite the nature of the work I do, and I passionately believe everyone can have incredible spiritual experiences. In order to aid you in having your own experiences, my main spirit guide, White Feather (who acts as spokesperson for the team in the spirit world who work with me), asked me to share the teachings they bring to you in this book in my everyday, down-to-earth manner and to speak in simple terms. The spirits relay that this will support you in learning to access a connection with the spiritual dimensions and your own soul for yourself.

There are many ways to unlock that doorway to eternity within yourself, of course, but to highlight the power of spiritual experience through the practice of evidence-based mediumship (one of the ways I help people unlock that doorway), the following is an account of a message relayed from a spirit father to his son. It represents well the message I bring – that the soul is real, and upon physical death we simply move into a spiritual body and journey on within the dimensions of the spirit world. It also highlights the eternal strength of soul connections, and emphasizes that, even after death, we don't have to feel completely separated from those we love. Death certainly ends the life of a physical body, but it does not end relationships or our soul connections. We carry those we love within our heart and soul forever, until we meet again.

3

DAVE'S STORY

Claire's ability to communicate with those in the afterlife is remarkable. I had been hoping she would be able to communicate with my dad, who had passed away suddenly a few years before. My mate had received a reading from Claire a few years back, so when he recommended her to me, I thought I had nothing to lose. I wasn't sure it would be possible as I know you can't call up the dead on request, but I did send out a quiet request to my dad to reach out to me through Claire if he could, and I didn't leave disappointed.

Dad came straight through Claire loud and clear. She described how he looked in accurate detail, telling me not only how he looked before he died, but also telling me Dad was showing himself to her now looking fit and well and in a younger spirit body. She described a photo I have of my old man when he was young. She could not have described his personality any more accurately either. She had Dad's great sense of humour down pat. She said he would do anything for anyone too, but he was also not an easy man to deal with at times and was stubborn. Her tactful honesty in her description of him was refreshing.

Dad died of a heart attack suddenly at the age of 60, and I never had a chance to say goodbye. Claire was able to tell me what had happened to Dad that day, including where he was when he died and how it happened. He had collapsed at work. Dad was a plumber and always doing strenuous work, and it was really hot that day. It must have been too much.

She also told me about a tattoo I'd had done in memory of Dad. Dad and I shared a love of reptiles, and Claire said she could see two snakes – exactly my tattoo in memory of him.

YOU ARE AN ETERNAL SOUL

> *To me, this proved Dad was still around. Only he would understand the relevance of those snakes.*
>
> *I've had so much peace of mind since seeing Claire. I know I'll see Dad again, so even though I couldn't say goodbye I will have a chance to say hello to my old man again one day.*

The spirit guides teach that the time to become soul aware is now. No matter how your life manifests in the physical world, and the challenges you face, you can learn to appreciate those challenges for the soul growth they encourage. You can access deep inner states of peace even in times of loss and sadness because you understand your own eternal soul. We are all souls, and my work is about giving people a glimpse of what may be possible in order to empower you to explore your own potential. You have the power to unlock within you the doorway to eternity and heal from the power of pure soul love.

The soul perspective

The happy benefit of being a medium who can perceive souls in the spirit world is that I have learned to view life from a wider perspective – the soul perspective. I have delivered thousands of readings throughout my lifetime to those in this world seeking understanding about the afterlife. During sessions, I have not only been shown visions of what life is like for those residing in the spirit world, but I have also been able to provide information to my clients that I could not possibly have known in advance, thereby providing personal evidence that the soul is eternal.

One example is when I connected to the spirit world for my client, Oscar. His partner, Leon (now in the spirit world), communicated to me that he was residing in a white lodge surrounded by heavenly scenery and free from the pain of the cancer that ended his physical life. Leon added that he was reunited in the afterlife with his beloved dogs, and also relayed that he visited Oscar regularly to watch over him. He expressed how much he missed Oscar and loved him still, and communicated that he would wait for Oscar in the spirit world. Leon then relayed to me that he knew Oscar had carried his ashes with him everywhere since his death. My client was amazed, and so was I when Oscar leaned back on the sofa and pulled a tiny bag of his partner's ashes out of his jeans pocket! Oscar then told me that before Leon became ill, they would regularly visit a lake in England that they loved, and stay in a log cabin with their dogs. Oscar explained it was their idea of heaven, and he told me tearfully that the information provided had given him all the proof he ever needed to believe in an afterlife. I, of course, found the pure soul love still shared between these Romantic Soulmates (despite separation because of physical death) very touching.

I think many will understand the benefit of receiving this kind of comforting information from a medium when someone is struggling with the bereavement of a loved one and how it can help emotionally. However, the spirit guides who work with my mediumship ability no longer limit their teachings to purely evidence-based messages for those who are bereaved. Knowledge of the afterlife being real and the soul eternal is just the tip of the iceberg as far as they are concerned. They also want to help everyone to see from the soul perspective, making greater sense of the challenges they face (including painful relationships and difficult life circumstances), as well as bringing soul wisdom to empower us to live more fully. As a result, the spirit guides who work with me began to lead those in need of soul guidance and healing to my practice.

Soul guidance and soul healing

In soul guidance and soul-healing sessions, clients attend in order to learn from their own spirit guides, as well as White Feather and the gang. In these sessions, the spirit guides not only connect my clients to the client's loved ones and ancestors, but they also give me insights into the client's life purpose by helping them to comprehend the soul lessons being learned in their personal life circumstances. In addition, the sessions provide a clearer understanding of the types of soul connections that occur in people's significant relationships. It is marvellous to know that someone you love is well and waiting for you in the spirit world, but the wisdom the spirit guides are able to bring about a client's soul journey in this lifetime is just as transformative for my clients.

Jemima, a client I worked with recently, had experienced a terribly painful and sudden ending to a romantic relationship. This led to her experiencing ill health, a loss of income, and her house being sold against her wishes. Through their unwavering love, Jemima's spirit guides helped her to see via my mediumship that, despite her anger and frustration at how things were changing in her life at the time, she was actually working through circumstances that presented an opportunity for soul growth. This was a chance for her to recreate the life of her dreams. Jemima was helped to understand the soul connections in her own life and what had led her to the point of the relationship breakdown. She was taught about her need to embody more love of self, and guided on the power of loving others unconditionally. Jemima was also given insight into a past-life experience where she had suffered the trauma of losing her home. It was burned down after a violent domestic dispute in that lifetime, which sadly resulted in Jemima suffering a fatal illness. The spirit guides shone a light on the situation in Jemima's current life by helping her understand that she was unconsciously creating a similar situation in this lifetime in order to soul heal from the prior life experience and move forwards, liberated. Jemima took on board the wisdom shared in this soul-healing session and began the inner soul work necessary to empower herself. Within months, Jemima's health had improved significantly. She was able to work again and eventually moved to a seaside town, where she developed her passion for creating arts and crafts, and, in time, met a new romantic partner. Her life was unrecognizable from when she first found her way to me, and when I last spoke to Jemima she told me she was the most content she'd ever been. With time, patience and her absolute willingness to look at life from the soul perspective, Jemima had surrendered to what her soul was teaching her and could now see with hindsight that her prior pain had been the making of her.

DID YOU KNOW?
After-death communication

Research on the brains of mediums using psychometric and brain electrophysiology data, carried out in 2013 by Arnaud Delorme PhD (a CNRS principal investigator in Toulouse, France, and a faculty member at the University of California, San Diego, plus a scientist at the Institute of Noetic Sciences), "found suggestive that the impressions of communication with the deceased may be a distinct mental state in itself, distinct from ordinary thinking or imagination". In other words, while the mediums were in communication with the deceased, their brains functioned in a manner not usually demonstrated by the brain during the use of imagination or ordinary thinking. This research suggests that mediums achieve a method of communication distinct in its own right and unique to the practice of mediumship. The finding is interesting because it helps rule out suggestions of fraudulence, as under test conditions the mediums were found to be providing information under test conditions not deduced by ordinary means.

Connecting to the spirit world to become soul aware

Working with the spirit guides to help people better understand their own soul and the soul connections they make with others is an aspect of mediumship and healing that I had overlooked for many years because I had placed an emphasis squarely on trying to provide evidence for consciousness surviving physical death and for the afterlife being real. The spirit guides, however, encouraged me to move my own understanding of the soul on, and, in doing so, evolved my practice and teachings too. They demonstrated pure love whilst helping people gain soul awareness, soul wisdom and a greater understanding of soul connection. As a result, I am now able to share what I've learned from them with you. I know they wish for you to be able to walk in greater soul awareness through life – to live more fearlessly, love more unconditionally and aspire to reach your fullest potential. That journey begins with my teaching that you are not just a physical being, or even a spirit being, but that you are an eternal soul.

Three is a magic number

As the song – written by Bob Dorough and then rapped by 1980s hip-hop group De La Soul (apt name for a band mentioned in this book, by the way) goes – "Three is a magic number".

Why do I say this? It is because we are all a tri-part being. You *have* a **physical body** and you *have* a **spiritual body**, but you *are* also a **soul**. Some might call this is a holy trinity, I prefer the word "triune" (meaning "three in one").

These three elements have individual functions but are interconnected, creating one whole being. The soul is primary in this equation, because to have any kind of conscious experience, the soul must be present. The soul is pure conscious awareness; the two other aspects of self (physical body and spiritual body) are mere shells without it.

When the soul leaves the physical body, it leaves behind a corpse. We all recognize this, especially when we see a loved one die and experience that sense of their animated presence (or soul) having left their body. It's amazing how the body of someone you have known and loved so well can still be there in the room with you, but you now feel somehow detached. That's because you are soul bonded, not physically bonded, and you subconsciously recognize the soul of your loved one is no longer inhabiting the body lying there.

You also have a spiritual body. This is an exact mirror image of your physical body, but consists purely of light. (Think of the translucent image you might expect to see if you saw an apparition of a spirit being.) The soul can shed this spiritual body too if it should so choose, and exist instead as pure light source without form. (Think of orbs of light, to understand what I mean.) So, although the soul can choose to take on a physical body and a spiritual body, it doesn't have to. In essence, the physical body and spiritual body are avatars for the soul. This is why I'm stressing to you that you *have* a physical body and you *have* a spiritual body, but you *are* a soul.

CALL TO ACTION: Connect to your soul

The heart is a portal to your soul. It has the most powerful source of electromagnetic energy in the body, expanding out ward from you by about 3 ft (1 m). When you focus your attention on your heart and learn to expand your own electromagnetic energy field, you tap into the unconditional loving power of your own soul. Do the following exercise regularly to bring your mind into alignment with your soul and tap consciously into its power.

1. Close your eyes, take a deep breath and still your mind. Let go of any thoughts of the day. You are going to connect to your soul via your heart.
2. Think of someone you love spending time with and the joy you get when you do (this might even be a pet). If you prefer to think of a pastime you absolutely love, do that instead. As you hold the memory, observe the wonderful feeling of love that begins to swell in the centre of your chest.
3. Place your right hand on your heart. This is the hand that represents giving. By placing it here, you bring more of what you need to you – in this case, love. Love is an energy that flows through you, so breathe in slowly and deeply as you focus your mind on the someone or something you love. Allow the emotion to grow and expand within you. Breathe the emotion in, like you do oxygen. Then imagine the energy of your heart expanding right out into the room around you. Focus on feeling the emotion instead of thinking about the memory you selected. Let go of all thought and just be with this divine power. Notice you *are* the love you feel. There is no separating your soul from the emotion.

4. Now repeat your slow deep breaths three more times and, with each in-breath, feel the love continue to grow and expand within you. You may smile as the feel-good chemicals called endorphins naturally release in your brain. Be still. Just sit with that love. Your soul is unconditionally loving.

Spirit or ghost?

Contradictory to what many believe, ghosts are not the same as spirit beings, even though a ghost may look exactly like a spirit being when sighted. The distinction? As mentioned above, a spirit being has a spiritual body and, most importantly, a soul. It is therefore able to consciously interact with a person; but should you try to interact with a ghost, you will not be able to because it does not have a conscious soul animating it. It will seem to ignore you completely, oblivious to your presence – precisely because it doesn't have soul awareness. Ghosts are simply a "recording" in the atmosphere of an event in time. For example, there are numerous records of the common apparition of a ghostly battle. Many report seeing soldiers fighting bloody wars in fields across the countryside, and these sightings are often seen playing out time and time again (usually on the anniversary of a particular gruesome event in history, as if trapped in time). Look up the fascinating reports of the English Civil War battle that took place at Edgehill – is the only ghost sighting to be officially recognized by the British Public Record Office.

It's the soul that really counts

It's funny, we tend to think of the spirit world as a world without form because it is invisible to the naked eye for the most part; but because people see apparitions, we can realize the spirit world is actually a world of form too (whether that realization comes from the sightings of ghosts or spirit beings). The spirit world simply takes a different form to our own physical world of dense matter, but anything that takes form (in both this world and the spirit world) is always temporary in nature. The soul, on the other hand, is indestructible awareness and permanent. It permeates the spiritual and the physical. It is therefore the soul that counts, because it is ever present in both realities and is truly eternal.

A spirit loved one (being an eternal soul) may therefore communicate to a medium, passing on information about themselves such as the conditions around how they died. The medium may then be able to ask further questions about that passing and the spirit loved one can answer. The spirit communicator may also be keen to provide information that shows their loved ones here that they are very much "alive" and well on the other side. They often relay messages of love and support; and if you are really lucky, you may also be able to ask that spirit communicator to produce physical phenomena as proof of their presence in the room with you. For example, the spirit being may be able to tap on a table, play with the lights or even roll a marble toward you.

I have personally witnessed all of these types of interactions from spirit beings, and much more. During readings, spirit communicators commonly show themselves to me looking really well and much as they did in their earthly lifetimes, but often much younger and in their prime. In fact, the spirit guides teach me that their world is more real to them than our own is to us. This is because they are able to enjoy a heightened experience of reality, due to the spiritual body not holding the same limitations for the soul as the physical body must.

Signs and indications your loved ones in the spirit world walk with you still (this list is not exhaustive)

- You feel their presence and a sense of calm and peace wash over you.
- You see them in vivid dreams where they look well and they relay their emotions to you.
- You smell a familiar scent or perfume only relatable to that specific loved one.
- You randomly hear a song or piece of music that is specific to this person.
- You see signs, such as feathers, robins, butterflies, rainbows, flowers or any manner of signs that remind you instantly of your loved one and then you feel or remember their love.
- You experience electrical activity, such as lights turning on or off on their own, the television changing channels to a programme that your loved one liked, or the doorbell rings and no-one is there, etc.
- You see them in meditation and feel their love washing over you.
- Their name appears in unusual places and maybe just when you were thinking about them.
- You hear their voice in your mind communicating to you.
- You visit a medium and receive evidence of their survival.

DID YOU KNOW? What we see

The human body must filter out, by necessity, much of the reality around it in order to avoid becoming damaged, overstimulated or overwhelmed. For example, the human eye can only see a small portion of the electromagnetic field and the total light source available in the universe (typically between 380 to 700 nanometers, or less than 1 per cent of the spectrum), whereas the spiritual body has no such issue. As a result, spirit communicators often show me that the spirit realms consist of the most beautiful colours and sounds. They say it is our world that they view as the dream world and "illusory", and this certainly seems to corroborate with the stories we hear from those who have had a near death experience (NDE). Neurosurgeon Dr Eben Alexander wrote in his book, *Proof of Heaven*, about the spiritual dimensions he travelled through during his NDE and their amazing beauty. This was all while his physical body was medically brain-dead and he lay in a coma.

Seeing yourself as an energy being

It can be difficult to grasp the concept that you are a tri-part being – a soul with a body, not a body with a soul. It's obviously so much easier to know yourself as a physical being because you see it with your own eyes, but this is actually the most temporary aspect of your "self". The physical body lasts a very short while – the blink of an eye – in comparison to the spiritual body, which has the capacity to last much longer in the dimensions of the spirit world.

Yet even your spiritual body may be dropped (or at least upgraded) by your soul at some point, should you choose. Your soul may favour a different identity from a different lifetime, or to exist almost entirely in pure soul light energy instead. This tends to happen once the soul reaches an ascended state of consciousness, where it truly understands that it does not need to identify with form at all because it is pure soul love, manifested from energy and light.

The soul can achieve this because, no matter the form (spiritual body or physical body), the building blocks of it all – absolutely everything in reality – is energy. As genius inventor, engineer and physicist Nikola Tesla put it, "if you want to find the secrets of the universe, think in terms of energy, frequency and vibration". Science proved long ago that everything is energy. The "law of conservation", first proposed and tested by Émilie du Châtelet, states that the total energy of an isolated system remains constant. This means that energy can neither be created or destroyed – energy just is. And if energy just is and always will be, then it stands to reason that you too, being very much part of the universe, must also abide by this natural law.

What's more, all energy within the universe is in a constant process of recycling. We see this with our own eyes – think of the change of seasons, for example, or how water turns from ice to liquid then to steam. The universe is cyclical and, as a part of the universe, you must be cyclical in nature too. You know you are. Look at how your skin cells shed and replenish as a perfect example. And it's not just your skin cells either – most living cells in your body recycle. In a literal sense, you are not the same body that you were as a child. Yet you feel you are, because the ever present indestructible aspect of you has always been your eternal and aware soul self.

DID YOU KNOW? The subtle energy body and the soul data field

The physical body is surrounded by its own field of energy which connects the soul to both the physical and spiritual dimensions. Traditionally known as the "aura", this energy field is also known by energy healers and spiritual practitioners as the "subtle energy body". Those who have developed the extra sensory perception of clairvoyance ("clair" meaning "clear" and "voyant" meaning "seeing") and clairsentience ("sentience" meaning "sensing") can perceive the subtle energy body as a field of colour, waves of energy and vibrating frequencies. If you could see the aura, you would see it as a torus (donut-shaped) field of energy, radiating light through the core of the human body as well as out of and around it. (It may help to imagine a donut-shaped field of light with a human body placed in the "hole" in the middle.) The spirit guides tell me that the torus field of the subtle energy body acts as your "soul data field", recording within it every life experience you have ever had in this lifetime and allowing the soul to retain what the brain cannot. How cool is that?

What's more, given that the subtle energy body's torus field of energy is a mass of colourful light, and light consists of photons (packets of quantum light particles), the torus field of the subtle energy body is also electromagnetic (electric light and magnetic force) in nature. This electromagnetic data field varies in colour and vitality from person to person on any given day, based on physical health, mental well-being and the degree to which a soul has reached a level of spiritual maturity and enlightenment. Can you begin now to realize how amazing you are?

CALL TO ACTION: Look at people as souls and not bodies

Try to shift to the soul perspective to see other people as souls first and foremost, then as spiritual bodies and not just physical bodies. Look around you when you are out shopping, in a coffee shop or restaurant, or at work. Begin to understand that you are journeying with eternal souls, not just human beings. Even your beloved pets have souls. They too continue on after death into eternal life – they have awareness as well, after all.

Imagine all the colourful subtle energy bodies of light around you. Maybe you can sense where their energy fields touch or blend with your own energy field? Then, as you look, say to yourself, "Look at that person's soul conversing with the other person's soul". Do you get a sense of the surreal by doing this? Can you access the soul level of reality and shift your awareness? If you can, go deeper still. Can you sense how we are all one and the same at the ultimate level of reality? The energy source from which individual souls emerge also unifies them because they are all fundamentally from the one original soul source (we can call this source primordial – meaning "existing at the beginning, and the earliest stages of development"). This creates an "over-soul" field of soul energy, connecting us all.

I know it's a lot for the mind to grasp because it is almost indescribable, but don't give up. If you catch even a glimpse of this soul level of reality, you are truly on your way to gaining spiritual enlightenment. Play with this exercise. Have fun with becoming more soul aware.

SOUL LESSON ONE –
You Are An Eternal Soul

To summarize this first chapter, science cannot prove the soul's reality by measuring it with technology or mathematical equations, so we must look within ourselves to gain first-hand experience of the soul. You are a tri-part being – you *have* a physical body, you *have* a spiritual body but you *are* a soul. The soul is indestructible awareness and permanent.

Loved ones and spirit guides who reside in the spirit world provide evidence of the soul being eternal through spirit communication. They wait for us, because of the love shared and the soul connections formed, until we ourselves return as souls to our spiritual home – which some may call heaven, or the other side or the spirit world. In the meantime, they want us to know they are well and that they walk with us still.

The spirit guides teach the importance of becoming soul aware now, so you can gain greater inner peace despite any challenging life circumstances you may face. Your eternal soul knows life in the physical world includes suffering sometimes; but when you view life from a greater soul perspective, you learn to find the deeper soul purpose in that suffering, recognize the soul lessons being presented to you and use them to transform and evolve in spiritual maturity.

By learning to see yourself from your eternal soul perspective, you access a deeper soul wisdom to carry you through your soul journey here in this lifetime. When you do, you learn that all you ever truly need exists within you – your soul is what really counts.

"This life is but a brief tenure, one of many perspectives
a spirit must experience in the quest for eternity."
Brian Rathbone

Chapter Two

The Soul Is Love

"The soul has been given its own ears to hear things
that the mind does not understand"
Rumi

We shop for love on the internet these days. Love is sold as something we can "find" – as if it is hidden from us and we just need to search to get or buy it. I suppose in a sense it is, if you understand love only from the perspective of the mind and not from the soul. The truth is that love is something that you *are*. This is probably why it has a mystical quality that none of us can really put our finger on or define with words, because *love is the soul*.

The spirit guides teach that we all came here to realize this truth about ourselves. As an eternal soul, we are pure soul love at our core. Love, therefore, is the most natural state of being for your soul, and it is important to understand that love isn't simply an emotion. If everything in the universe is energy, frequency and waves (as taught in Chapter One), then love is the energy with which your soul resonates and vibrates. We don't need to search for love, *we attract love* – because we ourselves are this energy.

You will find yourself in soul connections throughout your lifetime, without seemingly having to "do" anything. Love is a state of "being" within yourself, not a state of "doing". This is why love seems to just happen. You may not mentally understand how or why you love a person so deeply above others, but it is with these special souls that bonds of love are formed, lasting beyond this one lifetime. In this chapter, I'm going to put it to you that most people do not understand they exchange the powerful energy of their soul with those they love. Nor do they understand how to express this energy as pure unconditional soul love. Instead, most people love from their minds and not from their souls. They love others with conditions and in fear, with the result that most people can't nurture their soul connections to their fullest potential.

We are all challenged by the soul connections in our lives, especially those where loss or grief is experienced. Pure soul love is at the root of all soul connections, and until you understand more about it, you will navigate your own relationships with varying degrees of suffering. Therefore, before I can delve into helping you identify your soul connections in life and explaining their purpose, I must first teach about the love that you are.

In this chapter, I will show that soul love is very different to the conditional love most of us experience and express in this world. Without proper investigation of soul love, you might assume you understand unconditional love already. You could even be tempted to flit past a chapter written about love. Pure soul love is something most people struggle with. I know this because love is *the number one reason* so many people seek out my services or read my books.

Pure soul love transcends your suffering

Having delivered so many messages from the spirit world, I see that most of us suffer in this world in relationships when we love from a point of fear and control. Perhaps you've experienced jealousy over a lover for example, for fear they may decide they prefer someone else's affections to yours, or perhaps you have tried to dissuade someone you love from doing something that you worry could take them away from you? Maybe a child wants to move abroad for example, or a partner wishes to take up a career or hobby that involves a dangerous pursuit? In contrast, pure soul love allows for total freedom and expression because it understands that love, which is also the soul, can't ultimately go anywhere or ever be lost.

The spirit guides embody pure soul love and demonstrate it through their teachings. They never judge, and they show no need for us to behave in a particular way for them to be happy within themselves. They love us, warts and all, no matter what. They show us too that if we learn to embody soul love in the physical world, we can form the most wonderful sacred soul connections, and life here can be enriched beyond measure to a point where we may feel bliss.

They also teach that even if you experience painful loss of love in your life because you may have loved or been loved from a place of fear, need and control, the soul learning gained from this experience leads you eventually ever closer toward the unconditional divine love that you are within your own soul. Nothing is ever lost. This is why all soul connections are hugely important. No matter the outcome in this world, soul connections are always sacred interactions at the soul level, as we take the soul lesson with us into the afterlife. Pure soul love transcends all fear, suffering and loss.

You are the love you seek

In this world, so few of us recognize that we are the love we seek from others because we do not recognize love is our own eternal soul. The pursuit of love becomes wholly about seeking love from outside of ourselves, instead of seeking connection within the soul. We are programmed with romantic ideas and stories about what love looks like through popular culture, fairy stories and social media ideals – more or less from birth – with storylines of self-sacrifice, neediness, ownership or co-dependency. The temptation is to believe that when people love, it is normal to behave this way. All of this behaviour falls into the bracket of "conditional" love – love born from expectations that we then project onto others. However, it is possible to love completely and purely without fear, attachment and suffering when, within your soul, you already realize *you* are the love you seek to experience with another. When two or more souls interact with each other from this point of understanding, the experience shared can be blissful. The experience shared becomes an experience of total "oneness" as the souls come together as one.

The importance of discovering your eternal soul self

In contrast, the majority of us feel a sense of separateness from one another, even when we love others deeply, because we don't yet fully understand the energy of the love that we are, nor do we understand the way that energy exchanges between souls and unites us. We often place our own happiness squarely on someone else's shoulders, asking them to constantly validate their love for us. For example, have you ever asked someone if they love you repeatedly in a relatively short space of time? Or, have you experienced annoyance or frustration that someone you love hasn't demonstrated sufficient loving gestures toward you, such as spending "enough" time with you or buying gifts to make you feel special, or providing public displays of affection? I am not saying these things are not important, but a need or requirement to see someone you love behave in a certain way in order for you to feel happy or secure stems from the unconscious belief deep down that you need that something or someone so you yourself will not be diminished and weakened. You try to control what you fear would damage you if lost. Soul love, however, can never be lost, and nor can your soul be weakened or destroyed. When you understand this, love liberates. We may become separated from somebody physically, but never at the soul level.

CALL TO ACTION: Exploring the energy of soul love

Here is an exercise to do alone or with someone you love to see if you can explore the energy of the love you are from the soul perspective. We cannot force others to want to become soul aware, so if the person you love is not ready to explore spirituality with you just yet, you don't have to tell them you are doing this – simply try this exercise quietly while sharing an everyday conversation. This exercise will also help you to learn to tune into your own soul more regularly.

1. Sitting opposite your loved one and a little distance away (3 ft/1 m or more), send your love across the room to them, visualizing them surrounded by and wrapped in the energy of your love. There is no need to speak while doing this.

2. Next, sense the energy in the room. Do you feel closer to your loved one even though you have physical distance between you? Can you feel the energetic soul connection? How does that energy look in your mind's eye? Can you see or sense colours? Can you feel how the energy can flow backward and forward between you? Do you feel a sense of peacefulness together and a shared sense of bonding? Can you sense that the love between you is not really physical? Sit for a few minutes and simply observe what it feels like to feel energetically connected to somebody at the soul level.

3. A fun thing to do next is to try this exercise when your loved one isn't with you. Imagine them there next to you and send your unconditional love as above. Wrap them in your soul energy. You may find your loved one surprises you. They may unconsciously recognize the love energy being sent and reach out to you in response, maybe calling or texting to say they've been thinking of you? Perhaps they will come home having bought you a gift or will simply say how much they love you when they see you next.

As you learn to view your relationship through the soul as well as the physical world with this person, you may experience telepathy with them. You might see with your mind's eye what they are doing, hear their voice talking or perceive other sounds happening around them, or sense their mood or emotions. You may be surprised to learn how connected you truly are with those you love.

This exercise can also be explored with those you love in the spirit world too. Maybe you'll sense their presence or see signs in response to you sending love. Or maybe you'll simply realize the energy bonds and the soul connection between you hasn't gone anywhere … even in death.

In time, as you become more aware of the soul energy exchange between yourself and other souls, you might sense the soul energy contracting as you or they pull soul energy away when you have a disagreement. Notice how this makes you feel. Pay attention to the fact your soul seeks unity. Relationships are as much about balancing the soul energy between the two of you as they are learning to communicate well or demonstrate physical affection.

You can learn to build trust in the love you share with those you love by exploring the energetic nature of the soul bond between you. Over time, you learn that you are never really separated, even when physically apart. Pure soul love unites.

Pure soul love is what it's all about

You may now understand a little better that when I talk of soul love in this chapter, I'm talking of an energy so powerful it is the most creative force in the universe. I don't wish for the word "love" to come across as fluffy and airy fairy, or be confused with the hopeless romantic's idea of love. Understanding pure soul love couldn't be more serious. Ask anyone who was not shown the love they rightly deserved as a child about the devastation it caused their soul (not just their mind and body); or ask someone about the soul wrench they feel following the loss of a child or Soulmate. They will tell you a part of themselves is now missing. What part, though, if not the soul? This is how serious and powerful soul love is.

The powerful source of soul energy houses the human body and, when energetically connected to another soul through the heart of the physical body, creates a powerful soul love exchange tethering the two together. This creates energetic soul bonds of love that keep those souls connected beyond space and time, even when the physical body dies.

We are conscious energy beings first and foremost (which is the soul), but we are not taught how to lead our lives in alignment with this powerful aspect of ourselves. It's why those in the spirit world reach out to us time and time again, trying to help alleviate heartache by showing us who we really are – eternally loving souls.

From the work I do as a medium, spiritual practitioner and teacher, I've come to believe there is only one question you will truly be interested in asking yourself when you pass from this world into the light realms of the spirit world. That question is, "*Did I embody and demonstrate the love* **I am** *well enough and to my fullest capacity?*" How do you feel when you read that question? …

Many people I know have willingly shut down their hearts in an attempt to protect themselves from suffering, but if love is the soul's measure of everything, is this truly wise? Clients often ask me if they are fulfilling their life purpose. If you often wonder the same, this question will go some way to helping you find the answer. We evolve together united by the universal power of love and the realization that its ever present power in our lives is heavenly. This understanding is yours to obtain, and this is why those who communicate from the spirit dimensions consistently teach that you are on a soul journey toward enlightenment. Your soul is guiding you ever back toward the light and the love of the energy that you are, deep within you. Pure divine soul love.

CALL TO ACTION: Who am I?

You are eternal. You are the awareness behind the "I am" of all you experience. This "you" cannot die, nor can those you love. This means you cannot lose the love you share with others either. Practise the below exercise as much as possible. Get to know yourself at the deeper soul level. When you do, not only will you be in touch with your own eternal soul self, but you'll find those souls you share pure soul love with and who are now in the spirit world are able to journey right by your side too.

1. Ask yourself this question, "Who am I?". Pause. Don't answer straight away. Sit with the question and reflect. Are you your name? Are you your body? Are you your heart, lungs, legs, etc? Are you your relationship and role to another person, for example a mother, a son, a friend? Are you your occupation? Are you the actions you take or the interests you take part in? Are you your achievements? At first, you may answer you are all of these, but go deeper and you will realize these are all aspects of life external to the real you. There is a deeper you.
2. Ask again, "Who … am … I?" Meditate on this. Repeat this question throughout your day.

   Did you find your answer mentally? Or did you experience the truth? When your thinking mind grasps that it cannot adequately describe who you are, yet you become aware of your deeper soul self at the same time, then you'll be closer to the soul truth, your eternal nature and all those you love.

A lighter approach to love

Because true soul connections don't behave in the manner in which most relationships form in life, we must learn to approach pure soul love in a lighter way. Usually when we meet people for the first time, we connect mentally or physically, not at the soul level. If we continue to get along well with each other, over a long period of time our love may grow and our souls unite. This occurs once trust is formed and commonalities are established. Where true soul connection occurs first, however, pure soul love is present right from the start: for example, a mother's unconditional love for her baby from the first cuddle, if not before. Romantic Soulmates might fall in love at first sight. Twin flames recognize the love that is shared between them as an immediate eternal bond. And Soul Family members can't actually remember a time when they didn't love one another.

Meeting somebody new and experiencing an instantaneous soul connection can be confusing. Most people feel they must earn the love they experience with another, especially if they are used to feeling secure in relationships where conditions are placed upon them as the norm. People have a hard time believing they are worthy of receiving such love and accepting they can't lose it. Often they go to a place of fear within themselves and worry about getting hurt. It is then that insecurities may be triggered, causing an imbalance in the relationship and the two individuals to behave in ways that may be hurtful to the other. Things get heavy between them. Love has a way of shining a light on all that we must heal within ourselves; and soul connections can become hugely challenging relationships for many people for this reason, unless we learn to love more lightly. When we learn to love without conditions and fear, the soul energy between people shifts, even attracting souls back together who previously separated when the time is right. And relationships heal, as Isla's story, below, perfectly highlights.

ISLA'S STORY

Toby and I met through mutual friends. There was instant chemistry between us, even our friends commented on it. I felt like I'd known Toby all my life and, although it scared me to admit it, I knew I was in love with him from very early on in our relationship. Conversation flowed effortlessly between us, we laughed all the time, and when I looked into his eyes I felt like I was in my safe space. He accepted me, and I him. It was a connection like I'd never known before, and despite my reservations about entering into a relationship and getting hurt again, I fell in love hard and fast. It wasn't really a choice to make – the love was just there – and it felt scary to be out of control with my emotions in this way. Toby felt the same depth of love for me too, although he dealt with it differently. He was the first to say "I love you", and he talked from the start as though I was in his future.

Looking back, I had no reason to doubt Toby's love for me, but even so I did. I grew insecure over time; I think this was because I could tell this love was different and I'd be really affected if I lost it. It seemed too good to be true, to be honest. My parents divorced when I was a child and I had seen how bad things can get between people. My ex-partner had been deceitful, and I had been unfaithful in a relationship before that. I guess I had no faith in love lasting, and I measured my relationship with Toby against relationships in the past.

Toby was confident about us from the start, and as time went on, he was eager and willing to go to the next level. He was the first to suggest that we move in together, but from here things fell apart. I see now, in hindsight, that as soon as we committed to living together I became fearful of losing everything. If Toby went out with his mates and left me behind, I grew suspicious. Why was he so late? Who was he with? What if he met someone else? Why didn't he just want to spend time with me, like I did him? If Toby didn't send me emojis telling me he loved me while he was at work, I wondered why he hadn't been in touch all day.

I began withholding my affection if I felt Toby wasn't showing me love the way I needed him to. It was an effort to show him how he was making me feel. We argued a lot too because Toby was building his business and went away for weekends sometimes. He began to resent me asking for more time with him, and actually began going out more. Things became heavy and I shut down my heart, becoming distant. Eventually, Toby told me he needed a break from the relationship. When he moved back in with his parents, I was devastated. I began watching Toby's social media all the time, and sent him frequent messages telling him I couldn't live without him, and please could we just meet up. He didn't reply.

Sadly, a year before, my Nanna had died, which led me to booking an appointment for a soul guidance reading with Claire, and I had been waiting to see her. My appointment date arrived just one month after Toby moved out. At the session, Nanna came straight through. Claire told me all about Nanna's passing and gave me the most accurate details about Nanna's personality, even describing the little wink she always gave. It was surreal, and so comforting to know Nanna was watching over me. Claire then stunned me when she told me Nanna knew about my recent heartbreak and was hugging me.

Claire connected with the spirit guides at this point and gave me the most wonderful insight into the nature of my relationship with Toby. Claire explained about soul connection and what I was now learning from the experience. She also helped me to see how fear had controlled my behaviour and that my mind had deliberately sabotaged the love we shared. This was a shock. It was hard to realize within myself that what I thought had been loving behaviour on my behalf hadn't been love at all. The spirit guides talked of the love always being there with Toby and I, and they helped me to see the difference of loving freely without condition. They told me to take it lightly with Toby, to find it within me that if Toby didn't come back, I'd be okay with that decision because it meant I was loving Toby in the most beautiful way a person can love.

Nanna enforced upon me that love is real, and she told Claire to tell me that I must remember true love, like hers, can never be lost. After this session, I vowed to make a change. I stopped messaging Toby and decided to work on my own mindset instead. Loving Toby from a distance, I began to see the break-up as a blessing. It was really hard, but slowly I began to heal emotionally and to feel positive about life once more. I focused instead on my own spirituality, attending workshops run by Claire. I began seeing friends more, took up an interest in photography, as well as taking better care of my health. I felt a positive shift in me.

Then the most amazing thing happened. Toby reached out. He said he'd had a dream about me and he wanted to chat. That first call lasted hours. It was like when we first met. It was a reset. The chat turned into dates, and six months has now passed. Toby and I are back to enjoying time together and, without the previous pressure I placed on it, our relationship is doing great. We are both talking of future plans again, and I feel confident this time I can make it work. Claire, the spirit guides and my Nanna's love showed me that I was sweating the small stuff too much. Love, like life, should be enjoyable, and when it's not, it's not love. I'm full of hope now going forward.

CALL TO ACTION: Reflecting on soul love in your life

In order to embody pure soul love in our lives, we must learn to reflect on our own behaviours and bring conscious awareness to how we behave when loving others. The more soul love we can bring into our relationships, the more blissful an experience they become. Why not consider the painful or challenging relationships in your life now. Look through the list below and see how you might shift your perspective when navigating these relationships going forward? Can you see what your soul is trying to teach you? Next, think of a relationship in your life which brings you love and joy. Look through the list below again and see how many ways you are bringing soul love into that relationship already. Is there room for growth? This list is by no means exhaustive; maybe you can think of other ways pure soul love shows itself in your life.

Earthly Love	Soul Love
I love you because I get something out of it. You love me, so I feel good.	I love you and that love is given freely whether or not you love me freely in return.
I will show you my love as long as you behave how I expect you to.	I accept you fully as you are. The love in me is not reliant on your behaviour. Nor do I require an outcome.
I need you and I need you to need me too.	I don't need you to need me. I love you even if you don't need me. The love between us just is and will always be.

Earthly Love	Soul Love
I need you to act or look a certain way in order to be able to love you.	I am attracted to you inside and out. Your looks, age, social standing and gender have no bearings on my love.
I need to feel I'm special. I can heal your hurts and rescue you. Please do the same for me.	You commit to self-love and healing yourself because you love me, and I commit to self-love and healing myself because I love you.
I love you so much I would die for you. You can have all the love I can give at the expense of my own self-sacrifice.	Love cannot die. Our love is eternal. Love doesn't require sacrifice of the soul. It heals and lifts us up into higher love.
You make me so happy. Do I make you happy too?	I am happy within myself. I love it when you feel happy within yourself too. We can enjoy happiness together that way.
I feel jealous and threatened when others show you love because I could lose your attention.	I love that others show their love to you. I see why they love you. I also see it's good for you to enjoy healthy relationships with other people. I know you're learning and I want what's best for you.
I need to know our love will always stay the same.	I enjoy that our love is creative. I love the freedom you give me that allows me to grow.
You complete me. Do I complete you?	I am whole within myself and I love that you are whole within yourself too. Together we are wholeness shared.

Signs and indications you are connecting to your soul and living more soul aware (this list is not exhaustive)

- You can access within you a deep sense of inner peace, despite what may be unfolding in your outer life to cause you mental suffering.
- You calm your mind and become inspired, accessing your own inner wisdom and knowings, which guide your actions and move you forward in life.
- The hairs on your arms rise, or your head tingles as though your hair is standing on end, or you get the shivers when a new idea comes to you or you hear a truth that resonates with you. This response signals that your nervous system is responding to your subtle energy body while it accesses feedback and guidance from your soul.
- You walk away and can let go of opportunities readily that don't make you feel impassioned or just don't chime well with you, even if logically the mind is saying these opportunities make sense because they may be financially profitable, safe or risk-free.
- You understand you are not separate from anything. You wield the power of the universe and see through the illusion of death. You understand your indestructible nature.
- You learn to see the inner growth achieved from every hardship and relationship, then use it to allow the soul to elevate you. The paradox then becomes that suffering seems less of a hardship and you release it.

- You have a growing inner sense of needing freedom. You become more free spirited and start to dislike being controlled. You want to play and adventure more.
- You make time to withdraw from the overstimulation of a busy modern life and its mental dramas, and regularly choose to reconnect with nature in order to experience the inner joy and peace that arises within you from doing so.
- You are drawn to take up meditation and other activities that promote spiritual well-being.
- Your psychic senses become more heightened. You may experience prophetic dreams, for example, or experience gut awareness more often as your soul awareness emerges through your conscious thinking mind.
- You begin to see the deeper gains behind every experience in life and understand the soul lessons more quickly and readily. You notice you are able to release mental suffering sooner rather than later.
- You trust in life more. You feel confident to let your soul take the wheel and just go with the flow. You know your soul is guiding you perfectly and your thinking mind is not ultimately the power in control here.
- You begin to love others in total freedom, understanding that you are the love you seek and everything you need is already within you.

Soul merge and soul energy bonds

Emotions are the language of the soul, and it is at the heart that we feel the strongest connection to the primordial energy source that created our soul. Should we meet another with whom we resonate closely in soul energy and love, our subtle energy body, as well as our physical body, is attracted to that person like a magnet. This is due to both our physical and spiritual bodies consisting of electromagnetic fields. This attraction of electromagnetic energy forms an incredibly strong energetic "soul bond", which is why those who deeply love one another often comment they want to merge into one another, or they feel they can't get close enough to one another. The soul is seeking to become one unified energy force. Should you experience this sensation, this is known as a "soul merge".

On the flip side, when we lose love or are forced to separate from a soul that we love, we often say we are "broken-hearted". Even though the biological organ of our heart remains healthy, we recognize the physical sensations of the reversal of soul merge. An energetic disconnect (or unplugging) happens as the two souls, at the level of the subtle energy body and the physical body, pull away. We may even feel what is known as "core wound pain", which feels like actual physical pain even though there is nothing wrong with the physical body. This is because we are sensing the subtle energy body through the physical body. The human body is connected to the subtle energy body via energy connection points, or vortices, known by their Sanskrit name "chakras". At times of loss and grief, there is an unconscious recognition that the subtle energy bodies have become disconnected. This disconnection doesn't usually happen through choice. Soul separation is most often forced, and the experience becomes traumatic.

DID YOU KNOW? Earthly love vs soul love

To help differentiate and comprehend what "soul love" is, let's go back a few thousand years ... The Ancient Greeks were great philosophers and they identified eight different expressions of love, as they saw it. They called them:

- Eros (passionate sexual love and physical desire)
- Mania (obsessive, jealous, controlling, needy and co-dependent love with expectations)
- Ludus (playful or flirtatious with no commitment necessary)
- Philia (deep friendship, supportive, liked-minded love; you just get each other)
- Pragma (love that is pragmatic, withstanding the test of time and riding out difficulties)
- Storge (the love of family, including friends that feel like family)
- Philautia (self-love and taking an interest in self-care – not to be confused with narcissism)
- Agape (divine pure soul love, all-encompassing unconditional, spiritual love)

These days we only have one main word for love, which seems highly simplistic in comparison to the above. No doubt, as you read the above list, you can relate these types to at least a few relationships in your life.

Not all love is equal. We appear to love in degrees. The top three categories listed above are commonly transitory and fleeting, just like our earthly lives. For this reason, and for the purpose of writing a book about the soul, I am terming Eros, Mania and Ludus as earthly loves. These are often mind-led, fear-based loves, usually rooted in instinctual human need and ego rather than soul love.

The middle three – Philia (friendship), Pragma (long-term love), and Storge (family love) – are also earthly love because they are practical expressions of love that help us survive and thrive in this world. Furthermore, they are often rooted in conditions and a sense of duty. However, these loves also blend into pure soul love ultimately, because when relationships are healthy they demonstrate the wonderful qualities of unconditional love as well. It is these bonds of love that regularly continue with us into the spirit world and, because of this, mature into pure soul love. In the earthly world, these loves are balanced between mind and heart (ego and soul) and are hugely important experiences if we are going to live happily in a physical life.

The last two on the list – Philautia (self-love) and Agape (divine love) – are what I believe to be pure soul love. These are the loves where the thinking mind makes way for heart and soul to lead the way. These expressions are truly rooted in pure unconditional love and are not based on any earthly needs, demands or wants. If we manifest this love in our lives, it literally transcends this world and the experience is heavenly.

SOUL LESSON TWO – The Soul Is Love

Mother Theresa famously said, "*I have found the paradox that if you love until it hurts, there can be no more hurt, only more love*". She understood pure soul love.

In this chapter, I want you to better understand pure soul love and get the most from the soul connections in your own life. The soul is love, and love is an energy, not just an emotion. Souls share this energy, creating soul connections. Although most of us operate from a position of conditional love, the spirit guides teach us that relationships will challenge you until you can love from the soul, purely and in freedom. You learn to do this when you understand that you already are the love you seek from another. When you know this, you can learn to express the love you are with greater confidence and without fear, feeling secure in the realization that pure soul love never dies.

Pure soul love does not hurt; it is conditional love that regularly ends in tears. In this chapter, you are invited to imagine what it would be like in this world if more of us could embody the pure soul love that we are. You can learn to sit in the love that you are and realize that you, as an eternal soul, are enough.

"Ordinary love is selfish, darkly rooted in desires and satisfactions. Divine love is without condition, without boundary, without change. The flux of the human heart is gone forever at the transfixing touch of pure love."
Paramahansa Yogananda

Chapter Three

Souls Journey Together

"We are all just walking each other home."
Ram Dass

There is a beautiful serenity to learning to view all life from the higher perspective of the soul. What can go wrong, after all, if death is taken out of the equation? I'm not suggesting that your life is perfect, or that bad things don't happen to good people. People do make choices sometimes that affect both themselves and others in terrible ways. From the soul perspective, though, you can learn to find perfection even in the imperfection.

We cannot always see the bigger picture in life, so in this chapter I invite you to see from the wider soul perspective, and to consider that your soul may have chosen both your birth and your unique set of life circumstances (including key soul connections) *before* entering your human body. Awareness of this allows you to reflect upon your own soul purpose in this lifetime and consider why you journey here with the souls you do. Learning more about your own eternal soul will help you deepen your understanding of the importance of soul connections and pure soul love.

Souls journey together with purpose

Souls journey together *deliberately* with great purpose and meaning, reflecting back to each other what is not only needed for their own individual self-realization but, by extension, what is needed for all souls universally as a whole. This ensures every one of us has the opportunity to return to the pure energy source of divine soul love, when we are ready. For love, as I explained in Chapter Two, is what it's all about.

We don't endure the harsh reality of life alone, even if sometimes it feels like we do. We require the support of other souls in order to gain the most from the experience of life. We are all accompanied by fellow soul companions who have also chosen life in physical form at this time. The fact that you are reading this book is evidence that you are being supported by another soul right now, for example, as my own soul is guiding you through these pages.

Your spirit guides watch over your soul journey too, while your soul acts as the cox in the boat, steering you to the people and circumstances that will help you to create a life that holds deep soul purpose and meaning. The course of your life was set by your soul in advance, so in this lifetime it is now up to you to manage how well you row and align your oars with the cox's directions.

The astral dimensions of the spirit world

Have you ever found it curious that humans can be living on the same planet together and yet, for all intents and purposes, they experience life as if living in entirely different worlds, or even times? The same is true for the spiritual dimensions, where there are many worlds within worlds. Commonly termed as the astral dimensions ("astral" being derived from the Latin *astrum*, meaning star), it is within these dimensions that your soul first experienced soul awareness.

I'd like to teach you now a little about life in the astral dimensions, to help you consider that your soul existed before your birth and will continue to exist after your death. I have been shown that souls choose to enter into physical life purposefully, knowing they will meet with the souls of others with whom they already share a soul connection in the spirit world. It may be difficult to imagine and wrap your mind round some of what follows, but the purpose of me sharing this information is to better equip your understanding that there is a bigger picture and soul plan unfolding for you in this lifetime. Your life has great meaning and purpose, as do the soul connections you share with people in your life – which we will go on to explore in the chapters that follow.

With White Feather and the spirit guides for company, I have often viewed the astral dimensions clairvoyantly, observing that each dimension or realm is vastly different to an other, each serving different functions. These differences are largely due to the type of experience souls themselves create while residing there. White Feather tells me most souls choose to reside in the realms he calls "the Summerlands" (named as such because these are the realms where the light shines brightest between souls that exist together in loving harmony).

Previously, I explained that the subtle energy spiritual body is made of light and is a torus field of electromagnetism, creating a magnetic effect on souls, and just as you are attracted to people by their energy in this world, your soul would have been drawn to other souls in the astral dimensions resonating at a similar frequency to your own soul. I have been taught that when souls resonate at a similar vibration, the magnetism between souls forms clusters of souls, or "soul groups", and within those groups "soul families". This collective resonance is what makes the afterlife seem heavenly to the souls dwelling together in unity and love.

Spirit guides and the Summerlands

Spirit guides are souls that have walked the earthly path before. In doing so, they have now reached a level of spiritual progression that no longer requires them to be in human physical form. We all have spirit guides walking with us. As White Feather has shown me, while your soul was in the spiritual dimensions before entering into this life, your guides would have helped you prepare for the soul adventure you were about to embark on. They would have also teamed up with other spirit guides working to support the souls of those closely involved in joining you on this particular lifetime's soul journey.

You would also have met master teachers, angelic beings (powerful spiritual beings of pure love that have never been incarnate in physical form) and evolved souls who choose to form councils of light. The beings in the councils of light are so evolved in soul awareness and unconditional love that they exist as one collective, guiding the individual spirit guides on their soul missions and acting as a central point of wisdom for the benefit of all souls. Some of these ascended souls dwell in the highest astral dimensions of pure light and have no form at all (or not a form we would recognize form, anyway). These dimensions are often referred to in our world as the Devachanic planes in Theosophy, the heavenly realms in Christianity, Jannah or paradise in Islam, or loka in Hinduism.

Within the Summerlands, White Feather has shown me realms mostly consisting of natural scenic beauty, which really do look like the paradise we might expect from the most beautiful places on Earth. Only these realms are more colourful and vast, where everything seems to be vibrating with an aliveness we don't experience in the physical world. There are also areas with "cities" or "towns", where buildings radiate with light, as well as places that look so very familiar they virtually mirror our earthly world of schools, gardens and parks.

In contrast to these very earthly looking places, there are also dimensions within the Summerlands that look nothing like our world. I have seen beautiful crystalline structures that dazzle with the most vibrant colours and light. Plus, in the highest dimensions of the astral realms (highest because they vibrate with energy, light and love at such a high frequency, not because they are the highest in space), there are realms that take shape as simply pure frequency and light. These dimensions are beyond the Summerlands even, because they don't take form as we would recognize it. I can no more easily describe the scenes I've seen in the astral dimensions than I can describe cinnamon or honey with words. You will simply have to experience it for yourself one day. What I can say is that the little I have been shown by the spirit guides of both the Summerlands and the highest spiritual planes of light and consciousness in the astral dimensions is enough to ensure I do not fear death.

Every single family member I've ever communicated with in the spirit world on behalf of my clients has shown me they were embraced by the light when they crossed into the astral dimensions. They also relay they were met by loved ones as they transitioned, and that they are more than happy with their life now in the Summerlands. Therefore, as far as I'm concerned, there is no such thing as heaven and hell in the traditional sense. There are simply dimensions of differing resonance and a choice of experience. Love ensures your loved ones will be eagerly waiting for you on your return, as will your own spirit guides and helpers.

The guides reveal the "Before-Life"

In my previous book, *What the Dead is Dying To Teach Us*, I presented the case for reincarnation, and as part of this I also shared a personal story of what I believe to be one of my own past lives.

I recounted how, as a very young child, I had a lucid dream in which I experienced myself being stoned and forced into a pit full of snakes before dying from a snake bite. The dream ended with me experiencing a strange sense of emerging through darkness (like surfacing from deep water) before waking up.

This experience was completely puzzling because, as a pre-schooler, I had never been exposed to torture, the subject of dying, or watching films with snakes or similar content (these were the days of only three channels on the TV, and well before the internet). So, how was I able to have such a vivid experience of being utterly terrified before suffering the searing pain of stones hitting me and dying of a snake bite? What's more, the experience was so real to me that it left me with a fear of snakes and a memory that has haunted me to this day.

As well as sharing this story, I also cited evidence from scientific researchers who presented to the world hugely credible case studies of young children who remember past lives and whose stories could be factually corroborated. However, it's not just children that recall past lives. In addition to past-life memory cases, countless people across the world who have had an NDE have also shared stories of entering the light of the spirit world and reviewing their past lives. Psychologists, such as Dr Brien Weiss, have also shared their use of past-life regression techniques in therapy in order to heal clients suffering mental trauma due to past-life experiences. And, of course, there's also the information that mediums may receive from the spirit guides about the nature of past lives.

Pre-birth soul preparation

I have long since accepted the truth of reincarnation. This is because my own spirit teachers have often made reference to it, and because of my own recollection of a past-life memory. What's more, in preparation for writing this book, the spirit guides revealed even more to me about how the soul journeys through many lifetimes. As part of this learning, White Feather allowed me to receive deeper insight by helping me recall my own pre-birth experience.

My first insight was received in August 2021. While sitting in an altered state of consciousness for the development of trance mediumship, I felt White Feather draw close to me; then I felt as if I travelled away from my body and back to a time before I was born. I found myself standing in what I can only describe in earthly terms as a library – there were aisles of bookshelves filled with colourful books in a huge room. I knew this library was part of a much bigger learning establishment, like a spirit world university of sorts. I also knew this was where souls could go to continue to learn and educate themselves in the spirit world. I have since been told this "place" is commonly referred to as "The Halls of Learning".

While in this library, I was standing at a large table where a virtual model of the solar system was hovering over the table in mid-air. What struck me instantly was that I knew I was studying Earth in preparation for my return! As part of my study, I was familiarizing myself with the current times I was about to enter. I was also learning more about what I wished to achieve from the soul lessons I would experience here, as well as understanding I was being sent on a wider mission of service to others. What a thrilling discovery! I had no idea souls studied and prepared in advance for the life they would be entering. I'd always assumed the soul naturally gravitated toward the right set of circumstances it required; however, this vision implied I had intentional plans for my own incarnation.

What's more, as this vision played out, a spirit guide named Christopher, who I have been aware of for over a decade in my work as a medium, entered the library. What a revelation to discover I knew him before my birth! Christopher is a highly advanced soul, a spiritual master who often likes to take the appearance of an old-fashioned chemist or alchemist. In the vision, I could see that Christopher was directing me on the purpose and importance of the service that I was about to embark upon in this lifetime. The vision showed me that souls choose to journey together both in this life and the afterlife, and that there is purpose to every lifetime, even if it's not obvious to us while we are here.

Pre-birth soul memory

On a separate occasion, on 5 April 2022, I was woken in the middle of the night by White Feather standing next to my bed. This is something I've grown used to over the years, although it used to frighten me silly as a teenager. I now know that White

Feather visits in the night because it's often the time when my brain is most conducive to receiving what he needs to show me. At night, the human brain enters into deep (theta) brain wave patterns while asleep. For this reason, when waking from deep sleep, communication between the two worlds is often received at its most clearest. It's why many people experience vivid dreams of loved ones visiting them after they have died, telling them they are well and happy. These night visions are real communications of love, not just the brain processing grief.

On this occasion, White Feather communicated to me that he had broken my sleep because he wanted to show me how I entered into this lifetime. He made me aware I needed to be awake but also in a deeply relaxed state (hence the timing of his visit) in order for me to remember all that he would show me. He wanted me to be able to write down what was revealed, and then he made it known to me that the experience would be shared in a soul book I would go on to write. I get shivers writing these words now, because at the time I had no way of knowing that this book would even be written.

Because of the trust between us, I relaxed under White Feather's instruction and I was catapulted into what I can only describe as something similar to an out-of-body experience (except I also stayed aware of my physical body in my bed). I experienced my soul hurtling toward what I knew was the point of my conception, as if it was happening in real time.

It was the most surreal thing to experience. It was as if I was hurtling down a stream of energy toward Earth from a great distance. Within this stream, I was a point of attention. I had no body. I was pure soul, manifesting as a flash of conscious light, totally aware but without form, and being carried down through empty space in a stream of energy. There were no stars that

I could see. It was like a black void of nothingness, from which I was about to enter into a physical life experience. As pure soul, I travelled down toward this lifetime at immense speed, lightening quick. Like a shooting star.

What struck me most was the level of focus I was maintaining while travelling, and how utterly determined I was to make this journey. I knew that if I allowed my concentration to divert even a little bit, I could miss my "point of entry". I was completely clear on my purpose and why I was coming, and was utterly motivated to get on with it. I knew exactly what I was doing and where I was going, and I was also aware that, because I was descending from such a "distance" from Earth and at such a speed, I had to do this just right or another soul waiting to incarnate on Earth would be offered the chance for physical life in the human body that was earmarked for me. This was something I was not about to risk, as I knew there were others in my "Soul Family" (more on this in Chapter Four) who were depending on me to get this right. My failure to do so would impact upon the souls of those I knew and loved already here on Earth. They had signed up to this lifetime's journey with me and I wasn't about to let anybody down.

There was no awareness after that. Instead, I was back to full waking consciousness in my bed, sensing White Feather's guiding presence beside me and feeling his sense of joy in sharing such an insight with me.

Frustratingly, I wasn't shown my conception, so I'm not sure at what point my soul fully integrated with my baby body in the womb. I do know I have long carried a sense of homesickness within me in this life, as well as a sense of wistfulness and longing within my soul since a very young child. My soul is homesick for a homeland I have no conscious awareness of, but clearly my soul remembers. This homesickness has often made no logical sense given that I am not unhappy in life, so witnessing this vision and seeing I was carrying such a sense of purpose struck me instantly. My soul couldn't wait to get into this physical world. I vowed to remind myself to remember this vision the next time a bout of irrational homesickness arose within me. Here was my proof. I'd signed up to be here in this life. My life was purely my doing, and my responsibility.

Pre-birth soul memory validation

This story doesn't end here though, as White Feather had timed his nightly visit for optimum impact. After he departed from me, I jotted down the experience before going back to sleep. The following morning, a new client arrived at my door. Her name was Maria and she told me she had never received a reading from a medium previously, but before we started she wanted to reassure me that she already knew the spirit world existed. Maria then blew my mind as she began to describe to me the pre-birth memory that she herself holds. As I listened, I could not believe the incredible similarities to what I'd been shown by White Feather only a few hours before. It was now obvious that White Feather had chosen to show me this pre-birth vision deliberately that morning, before a client arrived who he knew would validate my own experience by sharing hers. In this dramatic fashion, White Feather ensured I paid attention to the soul lesson that I myself was receiving.

Maria has kindly agreed to share her story with you here in the hope it helps you to understand that we truly are all on an incredible soul journey together, here in human form.

MARIA'S STORY

I was four years old when I told my mother that I remembered being born. Unbeknown to me at that time, I was recalling the moment of my incarnation into this earthly dimension, which is something that most people can't remember. As you can imagine, my mother's reply was a sceptical one, and she said sharply, "Stop talking nonsense." Since then, I have never spoken about this with anyone else apart from two close friends.

I incarnated into this life the day my mother went into labour, hence why I said to her I could remember when I was born as I could recall travelling through the tunnel that connects Heaven to Earth, while being guided to this life by a wiser soul who was literally travelling behind me. I remember arriving at the hospital room and seeing my own mother in the bed surrounded by the doctors. Then it happened quickly and I entered into my body.

My understanding is that I was travelling to this earthly dimension through a tunnel that was dark. It felt that I was at a point where the lights stopped shining and I could only float (rather than walking with two legs because I was not in a physical body), then I started moving down in a stream and I could feel myself at speed, getting faster and faster. My very essence was as an energy being that emanated lots of light and, as odd as it might sound, I was not happy I had to come to this life. I remember letting this soul who was guiding me know I didn't want to come, but they said that I had to. I felt that I had no choice, and it was as though I knew I was entering into a life that would be hard and there would be suffering, which pretty much sums up what my life had been for quite some time, even at that early age. However, what has always struck me is that no matter how hard life can be, most human beings want to live in this physical world and don't want to die. However, back then I didn't want to enter here. I was sure there was something much more divine and peaceful where souls go when they pass away and do not wish to come to this world to experience suffering.

This memory or vivid dream I had didn't seem like a fantasy at all to me. It felt real, and it's still fresh in my mind more than 30 years later. The reality is that most people would think it was a fantasy or a dream that I had, based on things that I could have heard from other people or seen on TV; but how could I have acquired such knowledge about the afterlife/reincarnation at such a young age when my social life was nil and the only things I was allowed to watch on TV were cartoons? I hadn't even started kindergarten, didn't have any friends, nor was I left on my own with other adults.

I'm so happy to be able to share this very special and personal memory through Claire's book. This memory has been on my mind all my life and, for obvious reasons, I haven't been able to share it as openly as I'm doing now. It is fair to say that throughout my life I pondered sometimes whether it was actually a child's fantasy or not, but now I can say without a shadow of a doubt that it was a real memory, and that something much greater exists.

CALL TO ACTION: Connect with your soul self

We are all trying to remember who we are, and many people report a sense deep inside themselves of something missing or a sensation of feeling homesick. The soul knows the physical world is a temporary home. It is ever calling you back to the unconditional love you are within so that you can discover your unity with everything. When you feel lost, lonely or homesick for somewhere you can't quite remember, or when you have a sense of something missing from inside of you, use this exercise to bring yourself back to your true soul self and find inner peace within.

1. Light a candle. Look at the light and watch the flame. It is soothing to watch, and even hypnotic. Remind yourself that, at your core, you are this light too. You are from the light, and you will return to it.
2. Watch the flame and imagine its light filling your heart and cleansing away all heartache. Imagine your whole body now flooding with light – cleansing, healing and rejuvenating you.
3. Remind yourself you are not lost. Your spiritual home already surrounds you. Your soul is ever guiding you forward. Even in the imperfection, there is perfection. You are never alone and you are loved more than you know.
4. Sit in quiet reflection with the candle and play music that speaks to your soul. Relax the mind and see if you can just be with the candlelight, with no thoughts within you at all. Simply feel the inner peace within. This is soul work.

The science of pre-birth soul memory

Pre-birth memories are not often spoken about as openly as past-life memories. This may be because they are hard to verify, and so researchers have focused on the information given in past-life memories instead because they can verify certain facts, such as dates and family names, as well as the manner of death, in order to validate the memory being recalled.

Most impactful perhaps are the stories of young children recalling pre-birth memories, because young children provide facts that they shouldn't be able to know. One such example of this is the famous case of James Leininger, which was documented by renowned reincarnation researchers Dr Jim Tucker (child psychologist) and Carol Bowman. James, as a child, suffered nightmares while remembering a past life in which he recalled his death, trapped in a burning plane after crashing near Iwo Jima. He also remembered being based on a ship named *Natoma*, and having a friend called Jack Larsen. On investigation, the details he spoke about were found to closely match the life of James Huston Jr, an American pilot killed in action in March 1945.

Just as important though, is that in the process of remembering this past life, James also remembered pre-birth memories, describing what researchers refer to as the "intermission period" between lives. James told his father Bruce that he had picked him because he knew he would be a "good daddy". When his father quizzed him further, James said that he found his mother, Andrea, plus his father, Bruce, in Hawaii at the "big pink hotel". Bruce and Andrea had celebrated their fifth wedding anniversary in 1997 at the Royal Hawaiian Hotel (which was painted pink). This was five weeks prior to Andrea becoming pregnant with James. This was a fact James could not have known. This account adds validation to the spirit guides' teaching that we choose our life circumstances before birthing into this world. You can learn more details about this fascinating case of past-life and pre-birth memory by visiting https://psi-encyclopedia.spr.ac.uk/articles/james-leininger-reincarnation-case, or reading books authored by both the researchers and James's parents (listed in the Appendix).

DID YOU KNOW? Seeing your child before they are born

As further evidence that we sign up to our lifetimes before we are born, there have been many incidents where parents report seeing visions of their children *before* their child's conception. I have spoken to numerous clients over the years who have told me they dreamed of their child visiting them before they were conceived. I too have received messages many times from the spirit family members of my clients, telling me of babies that will be born here in this world in the near future. Plus, on carrying out research for this book, I came across this compelling account from Oscar-winning Hollywood actor, Richard Dreyfuss. Dreyfuss is one such parent who has been brave enough to publicly share that he believes he saw his daughter appear to him before she was conceived.

In an interview with Barbara Walters, the star of *Jaws* and *Close Encounters of the Third Kind*, Dreyfuss revealed that fame had taken its toll, and as a result, he had suffered from years of addiction to drugs and alcohol. The turning point for Dreyfuss to get clean came while he was hospitalized following a car accident in which he suffered minor injuries. He saw a young girl in a pink dress, horn-rimmed glasses and black patent shoes enter his hospital room. He told Walters that the girl spoke to him saying, "Daddy, I can't come to you until you come to me. Please straighten out your life so I can come."

Nobody else could see the girl, but the image stayed with Dreyfuss so strongly that he felt an inner knowing that if he continued on his downward path of addiction he would prevent this child from being born. He is quoted as saying in an article in *Mysterious Ways Magazine*, "I sobered up on November 19, 1982. My daughter was born November 19, 1983. My daughter wears horn-rimmed glasses. She wouldn't be caught dead in a pink dress, but it was my daughter, and the older she gets the more I see it."

CALL TO ACTION: Recalling your own pre-birth memory

If you would like to recall a pre-birth memory, try this exercise. Before you go to bed, ask your soul self to show you via your dreams a time before you were born. Set the intent and try to be specific. Ask to be shown where you existed before you were born into this lifetime. You could also ask to be shown why it is that you wanted to come here. Maybe you could ask who it is that you have come here to be with and why? Maybe your spirit guides can help you too? We often have to ask to receive.

Don't overthink it. Resist the urge to create a story in your mind. Instead, once you have asked, let your request go. Trust that your soul self and your spirit guides have heard your request. If it is in your highest interest, you will be shown something to let you know that you entered into this lifetime with great purpose.

Let your soul know that you are willing to receive insight in the form of a dream and that you wish to remember that dream when you awaken. Ask to be shown something that is helpful to you, something that will help you live your life in a more empowered manner, or give you better understanding as to why your life is as it is, right now.

Keep a pen and paper next to your bed. Should you wake up with insight, you can quickly jot down some notes before you forget.

Soul agreements are made with other souls in the spirit world

The spirit guides who walk with me teach that soul connections are most often agreed prior to entering into a physical lifetime. Maybe this is a reason why, for most people, deep soul connection remains a rare experience in a lifetime. It seems we choose the souls we journey with before we are born in order to journey together for specific purposes in a lifetime – both for the benefit of the individual souls involved and for the wider soul group collective. As part of this, we choose the key soul connections in our life, such as our parents and siblings in our childhood years, but we also agree in advance the significant relationships we will share in our adult years – many of which we know will be both nurturing and challenging in nature. To make it even more interesting, these soul connection agreements are often a result of shared past-life experiences together. This means soul connection agreements often span across several physical lifetimes. In this way, souls gain the optimum rounded experience from journeying together.

There are many types of soul connection agreements, each with specific soul dynamics offering different growth opportunities. All soul connections manifest in the material world in their own unique set of life circumstances because everyone's lives are different. Despite this, there are still common markers that allow us to identify the type of soul connection dynamic being experienced, and it's overriding purpose. I therefore share in the next chapters the most common soul connections that I see playing out in people's lives (observed through my own work with soul connections in my spiritual practice). I will also share the common signs and indicators of these soul connections, so you can reflect upon your own relationships and how you benefit from them in this lifetime. Most people don't realize soul connections have specific characteristics, but I see the same patterns playing out with clients repeatedly. In the work I do helping people understand their own soul connections and how to navigate them, my main aim is to support others in their healing so that they may gain peace of mind and come into wholeness within.

Signs and indications you have chosen your soul path before birth
(this list is not exhaustive)

- You developed a skill or interest at a young age that, on reflection, shaped your adult life. For example, you may have developed a passion and ability to play a musical instrument very well from an early age and so go on to be a successful musician in the adult years. Or you may have shown an early interest in animals and displayed a natural ability to relate well to them; you are now a vet, etc.
- You feel a deep sense that you are on a mission in life and must follow your calling. Even if you're not quite clear mentally what that calling is yet, you may recognize within you a feeling when you are going off track in your life.
- You meet someone and recognize deep down that you have met them for a reason. You have an inner soul recognition that you're supposed to be fostering this relationship, even if the reason for your meeting is not yet clear.

- You have been presented at times with serious challenges or losses in your life and, despite the suffering caused, you still feel that you wouldn't change a thing because you recognize the immense inner growth and strength you have gained. You know you are a better person because of this.
- Your childhood circumstances provided the perfect conditions to propel you forward as an adult. For example, perhaps a parent dies young of a heart condition, inspiring a child to work as an adult with the general public in order to help heal or improve the heart health of as many people as possible. Or a child grows up with financially poor parents, and seeing the suffering, limitations and sacrifices this involved, the child becomes an adult driven to build a successful career or run a successful business. With financial security secured, they now choose to give back and empower others.
- You experience dreams and visions of your life, or a sense at times that you've done this before and yet you can't fathom why or how you know that.
- As you look back on your life, you realize that everything came into place perfectly for you. The right people at the right time showed up, and opportunity presented itself with perfect timing.
- You recognize that when you have to work really hard for something and obstacles keep blocking your path, it's because there's something else you're meant to be doing or there's a different way. In contrast, when you're on track, everything slots into place fairly effortlessly; life flows with you and even unfolds in positive ways you could not have imagined.

- You have a nagging sense or desire to know if you're fulfilling your life purpose.

SOUL LESSON THREE –
Souls Journey Together

The spirit guides teach that you are an eternal soul that has chosen to enter into this lifetime because there are lessons and experiences you wish to master. Your soul resides in the spirit world between physical lifetimes, where you spend your time in heavenly realms within the astral dimensions, and here your soul continues to learn and evolve. When the time is right for you to enter into a physical lifetime, you agree to do so with other souls with whom you share a soul connection. No one journeys solo.

Souls support each other to learn soul lessons and evolve into ever higher states of soul awareness. These soul connections may have been established in other lifetimes too, in order for you to gain the greatest benefit from one another. Together, you soul journey and continue to learn from the experiences shared, supported by spirit guides and helpers who guide you on your spiritual pathway. They support you while you evolve in soul awareness in this world, because they know your soul is ever leading you back to the pure unconditional love within. You are never alone.

"Don't grieve. Anything you lose comes round
in another form."
Rumi

Chapter Four

Soul Family and Earth Family Connections

"The reason it hurts so much to separate is because our souls are connected."
Nicholas Sparks

As an eternal soul, you experience heavenly states of being when you vibrate in harmony and love with other souls. Your soul instinctively knows this and leads you toward other souls with whom you can share soul connection. Your soul strives for the experience of connection because it will lead you to the experience of love – love is the soul, and the soul is divine.

The paradox in our world is that many of us are not yet able to embody heavenly states of pure love. Seeing the eternal soul of someone you love, therefore, reflected back at you in soul connection is a powerful way to recognize the truth of your own eternal soul. For this reason, soul connections are the most impactful relationships in our lives. Your soul will guide you to both challenging and harmonious soul connections, in order for you to discover as much about who you are not (temporary, fearful and destructible) as to who you are (eternal, loving and indestructible).

In the following chapters, I help you to identify the different soul connections in your own life, and their purposes. I start here by teaching about **Soul Family** and **Earth Family**, and the differences between the two; as well as explaining why these connections can be highly challenging in their own ways. Soul Family and Earth Family form the foundations for many of the key soul lessons you face on your soul journey in this lifetime when it comes to relationships, and so are hugely important. We don't always experience every type of soul connection that exists in a lifetime, but we are almost certain to experience Soul Family or Earth Family dynamics in our lives, and often the two come together.

Your Soul Family

Your Soul Family are those souls within your soul group that, through common experience or shared interest, resonate so harmoniously in frequency with you that they blend ever closer to your soul – more so than those in your larger soul group. We term these souls "Soul Family", and these will likely be the souls you choose to incarnate into the physical world with many times over, because of the love shared between you. Soul Family connections are supportive, helping you to learn from all that life can show you within the security of knowing others will be there to help you along the way.

Soul Family members are the relationships we enjoy a deep and loving connection with, the people in our lives that just "get" us. Even if you are completely different in personality to other members of your Soul Family, you will still vibe high with them because you resonate together at the level of the soul (which is energy). Soul family connections largely make for joy-filled relationships. They are often playful and usually calm, even when disagreements happen or conflict occurs (because of course, we are still human at the end of the day, and no relationship is perfect in this world).

As an analogy, if we were to think of Soul Family as a group of different individual musical notes, these souls when played together would vibrate in such a manner that they would create a harmonious chord.

Within your Soul Family, you will also form soul connections that resonate so similarly to you in frequency that if we go back to the music analogy, these souls would be the same note as you, just on a different octave. These are our Soulmate connections. Within your Soul Family, it is Soulmates that usually come along less than a handful of times in a life. They are the souls that you would find it the hardest to live without in this world. Soulmates may incarnate as husbands or wives, biological twins or very close siblings, or lifelong best friends. You resonate so closely together that these are the souls we can most likely share heavenly experiences of pure soul love with. For that reason, they are also the soul connections we most often experience a sense of being "at one" with. I discuss Soulmates in greater depth in Chapter Six.

Finally, as part of your Soul Family but in a subcategory of its own, is also a soul sharing *exactly* the same soul frequency or soul blueprint as you. In the analogy of the musical notes, this soul doesn't vibrate in a harmonic chord with you (like Soul Family and Soulmates do), because this soul resonates as exactly the same musical soul note, on the same musical octave. If this soul played its note at the same time as you played yours, those listening would hear one note. We call these "Twin Souls" or "Twin Flames". This soul connection is greatly misunderstood, and the concept might even be new to you; I discuss this unique and powerful soul dynamic in greater depth in Chapter Seven.

Finally, I should explain that your Soul Family exists alongside other soul families within your larger soul group – just as your soul group exists alongside other soul groups. These united soul groups make up one infinite pool of souls in the form of one universal consciousness, of which you are an important part. Ralph Waldo Emerson (1803–1882), the American philosopher, poet, essayist and lecturer, named this unified collective grouping of soul groups as the "Over-Soul", a term that remains popular today.

Signs and indications of Soul Family connection

- You vibe high and spending time together is joyful.
- There is a deep sense of connection between you and an unspoken love that is simply an accepted given.
- You feel nurtured and supported – you can ask for advice and help should you need it and it will always be given.
- These are "your" people.
- Any disagreements are always worked through without damaging the love in the relationship.
- You have things in common or shared outlooks, morals and values.
- The idea of this person dying or leaving your life is something you don't ever want to consider.
- You choose to make time for each other and miss one another when you spend too much time apart.

- You feel a sense of security with them.
- Unconditional love is shared between you.

Soul Families vs Earth Families

I just explained that souls unite in the spirit world depending on how harmoniously they resonate energetically with one another, and that within your larger soul group there are other Soul Families existing alongside yours. Your soul may choose to incarnate into a biological Earth Family with souls from a different Soul Family to your own. You do this in order to benefit from the opportunities it creates – you can learn more sometimes from those who are different to you than when you only journey with souls that see from the same perspective as you do. When this occurs, it is commonly challenging because family members find it hard to relate well to one another. For example, soul learning is gained within Earth Family dynamics when you discover your Earth Family members are not those you turn to in life for support. They instead trigger you to foster independence and self-empowerment, because you must learn to stand on your own two feet. In this respect, Earth Family offer the opposite side of the coin in life experience to Soul Family.

It is common for Soul Family members to birth into the world at varying times to one another, and return to the spirit world in a staggered fashion. That way, there will always be Soul Family members on both sides of life, ready and able to offer support and love to one another. Soul Family members therefore might incarnate as friends, teachers, students, work colleagues or carers in this lifetime, as much as biological family members. Sometimes, a soul actually requests an Earth Family dynamic without any Soul Family members present for maximum soul growth opportunity. At other times, there may be both a mixture of Soul Family members and souls that are not Soul Family members in a biological family. Of course, sometimes a biological earth family will consist entirely of Soul Family members too; it depends on the best interests of both the individual souls and the collective. Earth Family dynamics are incredibly important because they allow for souls to interact with other souls from different soul groups and Soul Families, developing new connections over time.

Kofi's story below illustrates well what it's like to be born into a biological Earth Family while having no Soul Family members incarnate into the dynamic with you:

KOFI'S STORY

I always grew up feeling like I was on the outside of my family. My family is large. My mum and dad had five children, and our house was busy growing up. On the surface, life was typical family life. Yet, I could never find my place with any of my siblings. My eldest brother and two elder sisters are close. They were born five and seven years before my younger brother and I came along. They all married in their twenties and had their own families, which made my parents happy. When I left college, I wanted to travel the world – and I did. I have always been social. I didn't do great in school, but I've worked hard for years in catering, working my way across the world in various jobs, and I'm currently working for a well-known chain of restaurants.

I like my life. I've made great friends along the way who really feel more like family than my own family do now. I have a wonderful partner too. They are the ones who are there for me when I'm ill or lonely. My parents don't really get me, though I know they try. They openly let me know they don't agree with my life choices. They worry about my future, despite the fact I'm happy. I don't share the same spiritual outlook as them either, and sometimes I really do have to look at my parents and wonder how I ended up in this family. I don't see myself in any of them. They all seem to get along so much easier together than I have ever been able to get on with them. They understand each other, when I just don't get their actions or life choices.

I found this really hard growing up, but I'm learning to make my peace with it. When I saw Claire for a soul guidance reading after my close friend Mags died, Claire was able to explain my family dynamics to me. She explained that I had been birthed into a family who were not part of my immediate Soul Family, but that I'd come with the intention to learn from a different set of souls, and they from me, because this would challenge us all to open our minds and hearts in this world. It would help us all to progress. Claire told me we were being challenged to let go of expectations and love regardless, and she described the personal lessons involved for me, which I won't go into, but which were highly enlightening. The wisdom shared explained a lot. Claire described Mags to me perfectly too, explaining the soul bond between us and providing details of Mags passing and letting me know Mags is with me still. She even told me about the plans I have made for a celebration party in memory of Mags. No-one could know that. This experience has given me a level of peace and understanding I haven't had until now, and I'm really grateful for the teaching from Claire and her spirit guides.

The purpose of the Earth
Family only soul dynamic

Over the years, many people have come to my spiritual practice struggling with their family relationships. For souls such as Kofi, it can be hard to understand why they can't fit in with the biological family they are born into. They cannot understand, for example, why their parents don't seem to be able to demonstrate the depth of love they know they deserve, or why their siblings are completely out of reach despite there being no major bust-ups or family breakdowns between them. I can usually observe that the energetic soul bonds between Earth Family members that are not Soul Family members too are weak and distant. In fact, it's common for people to tell me that Earth Family members have drifted out of their lives completely. There seems to be nothing concrete holding these relationships together, and that's because the soul bonds connecting people are tenuous, or missing entirely.

These souls, biological family or not, simply don't resonate with each other; and, hard as they may try, they can't make it something that it is not. The lesson here is that everything is energy first and foremost in this universe. No matter if popular culture paints a rosy picture of what family life should look like, these souls are never going to form strong alliances. They came together precisely because their soul frequency is so opposing. We gain a wholly new perspective when we come to the understanding that family isn't dependent on the biological circumstances you are born into, and that love is not born from the physical body, but rather from the soul. In this way, souls experience a fantastic opportunity for soul growth and self-realization. Peace enters when we learn to see the immense opportunity for inner growth being presented to us from the challenges we face and in learning from these relationships – even if at times we learn the hard way. Among many other life lessons, such as self-reliance and self-dependence, you may even be forced to learn the value of boundary setting and self-love too. Try to bear in mind that it is not always your fault that things don't work out harmoniously in your Earth Family dynamic. Sometimes, despite our best efforts, the most loving thing to do is to create distance for a while, or even walk away until such a time that relations can be healed – if they can be healed.

If you are reading this and identify with Kofi's story, know it isn't because you are not worthy of love. You are in fact loved beyond measure. You have Soul Family around you, both on earth and in spirit, as well as spirit guides. Until your path crosses with Soul Family members in this world, strive to find love of self, assert boundaries and keep your distance from those that hurt you intentionally. Never settle for toxic behaviour or abuse, even from family members. Understand, if someone constantly criticises you, controls you, gaslights you or makes you live a life of fear, they are not your Soul Family. Earthly family dynamics often present some of the most difficult challenges we will ever be required to overcome, therefore seek out help from professional counsellors who may help you gain clarity of mind if you are really struggling.

CALL TO ACTION: Relating to difficult people/family

If you're having difficulty relating to family members, friends or colleagues who just don't understand you or who treat you in a way that makes you suffer, try relating to them at the soul level instead. Try this exercise.

1. We all recognise we have a voice within our own head that talks to us constantly. The voice in the head is our thinking mind talking to our soul self. At a time of conflict, go straight to observing the voice in your own head. Firstly, note what your voice in your head is saying to your soul. Can you observe your thoughts without judging them? Can you see the fear in your thoughts?

2. Now stand back from those thoughts. Breathe deeply and enter your soul space. Find peace within. If you can, are you now able to recognize the fear behind what this person is saying to you? Go deeper. Is there actually love driving their fear right now? If not, are you able to see how their own fears in life are hurting them more than you?

3. Next, remove their names or roles (Mum, Dad, sister, etc). Just be with this soul energy, as uncomfortable as it may feel, and particularly if it feels negative. Take a deep breath and in your mind quietly state, "This is your fear, not mine." Slowly blow out through the mouth and visualize sending their negative emotion back to them on your breath. You cleanse your own field by doing this and bring balance to the electromagnetic energy of your heart.

4. Next, imagine removing both your own and the other person's physical body. Imagine yourselves as spiritual light beings. Can you imagine yourself as transparent? If so, can you imagine their energy and anything hurtful they say passing straight through? Can you sit in your soul space and defuse the situation by becoming aware that no-one need hold any power over your own soul?

At first you may not be able to do this exercise until after an actual disagreement takes place. In time, you can learn to remain in your soul space and not get sucked in to fear and drama. It's not easy, but imagine how much better you'd feel even if you only achieved this 50 per cent of the time. Get good at this practice and you may even begin to see how much this family member has inadvertently empowered you. Then gratitude can follow for why you chose to journey in life with this soul. No-one can destroy or diminish you unless you allow them to. You are an eternal being.

Signs and indications of Earth Family dynamics

- You feel like the odd one out in the family.
- You just can't understand your relative/s at all, even if you try.
- The bonds of love between you feel weak or non-existent.
- You feel guilt that if a family member was to die, you know you wouldn't feel much grief.
- You may feel emotionally hurt that you haven't received the love you know you deserve.
- There could be toxic and abusive behaviour in the relationship.
- The saying "you choose your friends but you can't choose your family" is a truth for you.
- Your friends and pets are more like your family.
- There is distance between you emotionally, and often physically too.
- You rarely communicate, if at all.
- You would rather not turn to your family member/s for support and help, even if you had to.
- You don't trust them and you don't feel they have your back.

The Soul Family only connection

The opposite to the Earth Family dynamic that has no Soul Family members incarnate within it is the family that has only Soul Family members within it. Most of us incarnate into biological families that are a mixture of both Earth and Soul Family members. This provides balance in the form of fantastic opportunity for learning from souls that are different from us, along with the experience of supportive, unconditional love from Soul Family. However, some biological families consist purely of Soul Family members. This can be a truly wonderful experience in the physical world because the pure soul love shared is so heavenly.

Soul Families still incarnate as human beings on earth though, which isn't a walk in the park for anyone. It would be a mistake to assume that Soul Family incarnate in biological family dynamics equates to smooth and pain-free. We are all challenged in physical life and, whether we are with Soul Family members or not, we will be working through ancestral heritage, social conditioning, cultural ideology, world issues and the ego self. We will make mistakes because none of us are perfect. We will be triggered and challenged. Soul Family isn't about creating the perfect family experience, for that simply doesn't exist. It's about supporting one another while you do the inner work on your own soul journey to realizing your eternal soul self.

The purpose of Soul Family in earth family dynamics

Soul Family is about the degree to which we can bring unconditional pure soul love into this physical world and embody it. Even when you make mistakes or are hurtful unintentionally toward other Soul Family members, you learn that you are loved no matter what. In return, you offer the same loyalty to those in your Soul Family because you also love them unconditionally. This is the love that heals. Incarnating with Soul Family members as part of your biological family provides a nurturing environment in which you can learn important life lessons. Often, Soul Family in the same biological family experience massive physical challenges or loss. For example, a family member may have severe disabilities or health issues. Or, because they resonate together so well, family members may work together in business, which brings its own challenges – maybe a collapse of the family business occurs, or the loss of property. The challenge will require Soul Family members to pull together, no matter what. The emphasis could also be on collective experience and collective growth, not just an individual's soul evolution. In these instances, the challenges faced can be especially great, requiring Soul Family members to pull together as a team and to learn what it means to unite as a collective. This mirrors the way Soul Family exists in the spirit dimensions, as Olivia's story below highlights:

OLIVIA'S STORY

Mum and Dad were my life. As an only child, I grew up knowing I was loved completely. I was adored by both Mum and Dad. Sadly, Mum suffered a miscarriage a year after giving birth to me and it wasn't to be that I would ever have a sibling. As a result, my parents poured their affection on to me and also each other. We were so close, the three of us. I can honestly say arguments were a rare occurrence between my parents, despite the fact they ran the family business together. Life wasn't perfect, but it was perfect to me. I grew up in a harmonious home, where love and laughter were part of daily life. This was something I very much took for granted until Dad died out in the fields walking the dog one day. He'd suffered a brain embolism at the age of 48. I was 24 and his passing shook my world to its core. Mum had lost a doting partner, and I a loving protector. She was devastated, and in my attempt to make her world a better place, I put my own wants to one side.

I'd had no aspirations to work alongside Mum and Dad in their business, as I'd not long graduated in photography. Despite me having to put my dreams to one side and go home to Mum, it was still an easy decision for me to move in with her. Together, she and I helped each other through the dark days, and as a result, we grew ever closer for the experience. In time, we sold the holiday home Mum and Dad owned and Mum joined me in helping me to set up my own business. It didn't come easy, but we had each other for support and my mum was absolutely brilliant. She knew how to run a business and wasn't shy of hard work.

Over the next few years, I had a couple of long-term romantic relationships, but they never seemed to proceed to serious commitment and both ended in hurt. Deep down I couldn't leave Mum, so whoever dated me had to accept Mum in the equation. Our bond was unbreakable. When Mum was diagnosed with bowel cancer at the age of 60, I couldn't believe this was happening to me again. At 35, I was faced with the prospect of being alone in life and I was terrified. I had some great friends of course, but nothing as close as my relationship with my mum. No-one could replace her. She battled for five years and fought to stay with me. She was such an inspiration.

I nursed her at home until her final weeks, before she eventually passed away in hospital and joined my wonderful dad. I found myself rebuilding my life completely again at aged 40. With no husband or kids in my life for distraction, the grief was heavy. My parents were my Soul Family, and although I've recently met a wonderful man who has a big family of his own that I can enjoy being a part of, it's not the same and I miss my parents terribly. I feel absolutely lost in this world without them. Nothing can replace the closeness of love I shared with them, and although I'm grateful for what I have in life now (I know I'm one of the lucky ones), I can't help feeling orphaned, deep down. Mum and Dad, I want to tell you if you are watching me write this, how much I love you still. I watch for the signs you are with me. You were the most wonderful parents I could ever have asked for. I pray you're happy together in heaven and that I will see you again one day. I miss you, but I am so grateful for everything you gave me. You taught me the meaning of true love.

Olivia's story is a prime example of the circumstances that may manifest if a family consisting purely of Soul Family members incarnates here on Earth. The bonds shared are deeply loving and harmonious with rarely any discord, yet each soul still has ego mind and shadow work to do within themselves, in order to evolve in soul awareness. That's not to say that Soul Family members don't trigger each other, they do, but they often know how to forgive and forget because they understand their loved ones from a deeper soul level. The downside of Soul Family dynamics does tend to be that Soul Family members become extremely reliant on one another. Soul Family members are in their safe space with each other and often don't place deep trust in other souls so readily. This can mean they may live less adventurous lives, or hold themselves back from reaching their fullest potential, especially if they are not willing to expand out from the Soul Family group.

Friends and work companions outside of the group offer balance in the equation, because they are souls from wider soul groups. There is much to be gained from this and our lives become even more enriched when we reach out in connection and meet many different souls from different soul groups. The biggest downside to Soul Family comes when one or more Soul Family members transition back to spirit. For those left behind, the loss is crushing. The Soul Family members remaining here in physical life often report feeling that they no longer can find their place in the world. They long for unity back in the Soul Family collective in the spirit world. This will have to wait though, as they can't return to the astral dimensions of the spirit world until they have completed their reasons for being here. Their life here is not just about their Soul Family – to demonstrate love to souls outside the Soul Family is also important, as is being part of someone else's soul journey experience.

If you are reading this and you resonate with Olivia's story, and if you are feeling a lack of purpose or meaning since the loss of a Soul Family member, please take heart. You have experienced a depth of soul love not everyone experiences on Earth. Connect with your soul. Try to truly resonate with the fact your bonds extend beyond this world and find something you love to do in the meantime and meet others of a like mind. There could be more Soul Family members waiting in the wings to enter your life, or you could help others experience the love you were shown so they, in turn, embody love and pass it on. Your life has great meaning, and although it's tough when Soul Family members return to the spirit world, you have to remember that love never dies. It only deepens and purifies. You are not alone. Your loved ones walk with you still. You cannot be separated at the level of your soul. So, what will you do with the time you have on this planet without them? Live fully in honour of your loved ones and celebrate them by living well. Learn to go into your own soul. Feel the love in your heart. You carry your Soul Family members within you always.

Angel babies and the loss of a child

Arguably one of the most painful soul connections on this planet is the Angel baby/Angel child connection. These are souls who enter physical life for a short duration only, dying young. They do not stay long enough to become tainted by negativity in this world and remain pure of spirit. For this reason, they earn the title of "angel". I could not write about Soul Families without touching upon this particular connection and trying to bring some hope, because experiencing the unconditional nature of this love and the attachment it creates, then dealing with the subsequent physical separation and loss is monumental. I am not an expert in grief counselling, nor have I lost a child in this life. I am not in a position to say how a person should deal with the loss of a child, I can only compassionately offer the soul perspective in the hope it may shine some light in the darkness to all those suffering such intense pain.

I understand that the purer the depth of soul love we share with another, the greater the sense of loss there is going to be when we lose that soul from the physical world. For most parents, the love of their children eclipses all other loves they know, because for most parents it is the closest they get to giving another human being pure soul love. Even then, we still don't always manage to love our children as unconditionally as we may like. One of the greatest gifts of parenting though, is that we learn to become more compassionate human beings, expanding our heart-centred energy out into the world.

Mothers experience their subtle energy body blending with their baby's subtle energy body throughout pregnancy. The loss felt by most mothers when a child dies therefore, even as an older child, literally feels like a part of themselves has been wrenched away. This is because, energetically, mother and child were bonded so strongly on every level. The energetic separation that occurs as the two subtle energy bodies separate and the soul fields move apart can feel physically, emotionally and spiritually unbearable. The void left behind in the heart centre, no matter the age of the child, feels massive.

Let me not appear to leave out, or downgrade in any way, the pain a father feels at the loss of a child either. Dads are energetically connected through genes and DNA of course, which hold just as strong a soul connection tie. There are so many wonderfully loving fathers in this world who bond unconditionally with their children. I know, because I meet as many devastated fathers in my spiritual practice as I do mothers.

Finding meaning at the soul level

Many parents I meet are at a complete loss to understand why such a pure loving being as a child or baby must return to the spirit world so young. It seems so unfair. In addition, their hopes and dreams and life expectations for both their child and themselves are dashed. The death of a child is the ultimate in having to surrender to a greater power than ourselves, and become soul aware.

The truth is that souls don't always come into the physical form to live long lives here. Angel babies and children crack open the hearts of those around them in this lifetime, bringing soul love into embodiment in the world through their parents. It is usual for parents to tell me there was an ethereal quality about their angel child, and that they seemed like an old soul in a young body. These children touch everyone's hearts for the better in only a short time. To the soul, longevity of lifespan is not the purpose of being here. The parent and child will be reunited when the time is right. Until then, the parent now has the chance to reach inside themselves to find those eternal bonds carried forever in their heart and to use the pain they experience to become aware of the eternal nature of their own soul. As a parent myself, my heart goes out to all those who have loved and had to let go of their children in this world. These parents always amaze me with their strength of spirit and resilience. They are all inspirational master teachers in my eyes.

You will be together again

I bring a message of eternal life and hope. No matter how short a life in this physical world, there is always great meaning to it. Not only on an earthly level, but even more so spiritually speaking. Soul journeys are complex and multi-faceted. We have to look at them from a greater soul perspective or the harshness of physical life simply makes no sense at all. At the soul level, however, nothing is ever lost.

If souls choose their journeys, and children choose their parents, then angel babies and angel children specifically choose their parents because they know that parent can grow spiritually from the child's soul touching their life. They also know they are entering life with a higher calling at the soul level and that they will never truly be separated from that parent. They will see them again soon enough. Taking all this into consideration, transformation and soul healing may begin, as Sara's story honouring her angel son, Lucas, is a shining example of:

SARA'S STORY

On 6 September 2001, Lucas came into this world. On that morning, my world changed for the better. I finally felt whole, my life had a new purpose and meaning. The love that I felt as I looked at him was so powerful that in that moment nothing else existed or mattered – he was my whole world. It is the closest I have ever come to feeling unconditional love. I would have done anything to protect him as he was so vulnerable and needed me.

As a little one he was attached to my hip constantly. The world seemed to scare him, and it took Lucas a long time to find his confidence and his way. But my goodness he turned into an amazing young man – kind, caring, helpful, upbeat and trying to live life to the fullest. He tried so hard to make others happy and hid his own anxieties and worries; I couldn't have been more proud. He was literally one in a million. He taught me so much in life on how to love and I wouldn't have missed a moment.

On the morning of 6 November 2018, tragically Lucas was taken from us. As soon as I opened the door to the police officer I knew. I had received warnings as I had seen it in my dreams prior to that and I felt it in my heart, but I did not want the officer to say the words because that would be the end – no hope left.

My world shattered that day, my heart broke into a thousand pieces. The pain and heaviness in my heart was unbearable. I had no idea how I was going to carry on without Lucas. I blamed myself, the guilt of not protecting him consumed me. You are not supposed to out-live your child, you are supposed to protect them.

The worst part was he was alone when he died. Who was looking after him when I couldn't get to him and make it better? He was on his way to work and his bike hit gravel, which caused him to skid and he went under a quarry lorry. Thankfully, it was so quick he did not suffer. It was a tragic accident that should never have happened.

The following days were like living under a dark cloud of nothingness. I was living in limbo, waking each morning and being hit with the reality again. The pain was relentless. I felt so helpless. I can't remember how many days I cried for him.

I needed to check he was okay. Where was he? Was he okay? Then signs that we couldn't explain started. I began to smell him, feel his soul around me. "I" was written on the bonnet of the car randomly. He touched my arm and I felt it – it was a cold tingling sensation and extremely real. He appeared in my dreams, and I spoke to him constantly. He tried so hard to let us know he was safe, and I begged relatives in the spirit world to take good care of him because I couldn't any more. I couldn't stop being Mum – I needed to find out where he was. I felt it was time to see a medium.

I was sceptical at first, but the things the medium said left me with no doubt Lucas was still there around me and I wasn't *crazy. So a new journey began. I began to spiritually awaken. I joined a circle and started developing my own mediumship abilities, as I now knew Lucas was there. I meditated daily and read as many books as I could on the afterlife and mediumship, plus the near death experience. I joined spiritual awareness groups online – anything to get closer to him and understand what he was going through. I would have gone to the ends of the universe to find him. It was scary, frustrating and confusing, but I loved him and I wasn't going to give up.*

Throughout this time, he always found a way of letting me know he was safe and okay, but I felt I needed to see him myself. The only way was to develop my own connection to spirit and to go within to my own soul. Finally, the hard work and healing paid off as, 18 months later, Lucas appeared in my meditation. He looked amazing! So strong, so bright and so peaceful. He had grown. It was extremely emotional, but it was the proof I needed. In that moment I knew we would never truly be separated again.

I lost a huge part of myself the day Lucas was taken away, but I'm grateful for every day I had with him and now my spiritual path has given us a different way of being together. It will never be the same, but I know our love and bond is growing stronger each day. It still hurts terribly, but it's more bearable. My human mind may not remember all our meetings together but my heart and soul does.

I am the person I am today because of Lucas. It was an honour to be chosen as his Mum and I will continue to be so, just in a different way to what I wanted. That's the nature of unconditional love; it bends and where there is love, there is always hope. I have to take the long path, but I know I shall be back with him one day.

CALL TO ACTION:
Embodying the love you are

If you are reading this book wanting to make a soul connection in your own life, you should first become within yourself the love you seek from others. There are no short cuts or magic tricks to attracting a deep soul connection. They happen when the soul is ready, and they are always driven firstly by energetic attraction, not mental concepts and ideas.

Like attracts like. When you become the love you seek, you'll attract the same energy back to you. Do this by making time to do what you love. Get playful. Make time for fun. Take care of yourself like you would someone you love. Romance yourself even. Do this and you'll notice that, rather than you needing soul connection in your life, souls will now show up to simply add to the joy you're already experiencing. You won't expect anyone to provide you with what is missing in your life when you're already embodying all the love you need. Magically, when this occurs, you'll find love shining back to you from all the people you surround yourself with.

It is then that you'll understand it was never about finding "the one". As lovely as that idea is, it is still limited. It's about finding oneness within yourself and connection with all the souls that journey with you.

SOUL LESSON FOUR – Soul Family
and Earth Family Connections
Provide Soul Lesson Foundations

The spirit guides teach that there is a difference between Soul Family and biological Earth Family dynamics, and we learn so much from both. Soul Family members are the closest and most significant relationships in our lives. These supportive connections enrich our lives, and the bonds of love we share are eternal. We journey through life with our Soul Family members ever by our side, whether that is in physical form or when our beloved Soul Family members have returned to the spirit world. Soul Family are the souls within your soul group that, through common experience or shared interest, resonate so harmoniously in frequency with you.

In contrast, Earth Family members are often emotionally distant, non-supportive relationships, and may challenge us immensely. They force us to stand strong on our own feet and grow in self-reliance and self-resilience. We have to find the strength of our own soul within. We function materially with our Earth Family members, but we don't vibe high. They show us love is soul deep and not a physical phenomenon.

People in Earth Family dynamics may feel guilty because deep down they know that should an Earth Family member cross back to the spirit world, their grief would not be too traumatic. In contrast, our Soul Family members are the soul connections we would hate to live without. When a Soul Family member returns to the spirit world, the grief we experience is immense.

We must learn to search within ourselves for the love we share, to realize that because love (being soul energy and emotion) is not a physical thing, we can never lose the love we share with a Soul Family member. Love was never physical in the first place. Soul Family connections are eternal. You will see your loved ones again because love, like the soul, never dies.

"Some of the greatest battles will be fought within the silent chambers of your own soul."
Ezra Taft Benson

Chapter Five

Karmic and Catalyst
Soul Connections

*"Out of suffering have emerged the strongest souls;
the most massive characters are seared with scars."*
Kahlil Gibran

Most of us recognize that the experience of love in all its many expressions has the power to heal and make us whole, *if* we allow it. We all seek loving connection with others, and for many of us that includes those in this life and those we love in the afterlife too. Love is the driving force that leads us all to enlightenment, and this chapter explains the importance of learning to love yourself unconditionally and embodying the love that you are. The spirit guides themselves teach that until you learn to do this, you will experience both nurturing and painful soul connections as part of your soul journey. To help you understand this truth, I share information about two painful soul connections – the **Karmic** and the **Catalyst** soul connections. Although different in dynamics, both soul connections lead to greater unconditional self-love. Most of us are guilty of not loving ourselves wholly, and we learn painfully through these connections that we must not ignore the importance of self.

The spirit guides also show me that the purpose of both connections is to transform your thinking so you can let go of negative behaviour traits and the ideas that no longer serve your highest good. Spiritually, this is known as an "ego death".

In this chapter I help you to understand what an ego death is, as well as how to identify these karmic and catalyst soul connection dynamics in your own life. It is so important that we understand these two types of soul connections from the soul perspective – ignoring or refusing to accept the lessons your soul is trying to show you will only lead to you attracting more of the same experiences in life. That is, until you become ready to shift your thinking, reach for higher love within and become soul aware. When you learn to love yourself with all your soul, as unconditionally as you give love to others, you will heal emotionally; it is then you will appreciate that these unforgettable soul connections will have been a gift to you.

We get what we need, not what we want

Love is supposed to be a nurturing experience, one where we can feel safe and secure just for being who we are; but pure love can also trigger our insecurities and deep-rooted fears. This often brings out a side to our character we might not like much or may not have faced up to before, which can feel painful and overwhelming until we change our ways and heal. Within relationships, the love from another acts to reflect back to us (to varying degrees of intensity) the love that we are inside ourselves. The adage that you cannot truly love another until you love yourself first proves true, for if we are not in alignment with the pure soul love that we are, we will attract to us a soul that will behave in such a manner as to push us to go within to discover how strong we are, and to heal with self-love.

Even when a soul connection between two people extends beyond this one lifetime, their physical relationship in this lifetime could be short-lived and destructive – perhaps lasting only a few weeks or months before ending with a bang. This could be lovers that fall head over heels for each other only to be torn apart by family members against their will, or due to a conflict of interest or sense of duty. Or perhaps an intimate relationship between two people lasting longer (a few years even) which falls apart with an abrupt and painful ending – with one cheating on the other or being ditched at the altar. The truth is that we most often get what we need in life, not what we want. These relationships drive us deep within ourselves to find strength, courage, empowerment and wisdom, as well as demanding that we look at our own mental and emotional weaknesses and areas for growth.

Love's healing nature is therefore paradoxical, because although the experience of love can help us to ascend into expanded states of soul awareness, it is love itself that will likely bring us to our knees first, often in the form of a Karmic or Catalyst soul connection. Both connections require the letting go of ideas you hold about self, love and life that create suffering otherwise. They transform your mental perspective. In spiritual terms, this mental transformation is the "ego death", so let's learn more about this first.

The death of the ego

Ego death is exactly what it implies – the death of the egotistical self. Thoughts and ideas held in the mind and often programmed from young have to "die" to make way for a new level of enlightenment. The mind has to yield to a greater force – the soul.

Ego death is painful because it forces a person out of their comfort zone. Let me explain: imagine someone who has developed a deep-rooted fear of losing love, because when growing up, their parents didn't show them enough care or attention. As a child, this may have been interpreted internally as "I am not worthy of love". If this mindset is carried into adulthood, it can manifest as deep-rooted insecurity in romantic relationships, even causing separation anxiety. As a result, a person may show a need for continual affirmation of their being worthy of love, by seeking regular displays of affection from a romantic partner and becoming upset or anxious when this need isn't met. As wonderful as intimacy is in a relationship, if its underlying expression is not from love but from fear, it can become a destructive means to controlling another person. This may eventually create conflict in the relationship, making the partner feel smothered or trapped at the excessive neediness or jealousy, likely leading to anger, frustration and arguments. If the relationship then breaks down, the one with the deep-rooted belief that they are not worthy of love will have caused their own worst fear (loss of love) to manifest. Unless they now let love teach them what they need to change about themselves in order to release the ego mindset of "they are not worthy of love", the soul will likely draw to them the same soul connection dynamic again in the form of a different person. If this painful breakdown of their relationship teaches them to love themselves more by leading them to realize they are worthy of love and have always been, there will be a shift in perspective and a natural death of the ego occurs as they surrender to the heart and align with the soul instead.

Ego death hurts

Painful soul connections force us to face our fears and weaknesses, addressing jealousy, neediness, anger and so on. We learn to take responsibility for our mental well-being. Practices such as meditation help to still the mind, so we can find inner peace, step back and reflect. Speaking to ourselves in a more loving and encouraging manner helps too. We must take positive action, looking for a new perspective that brings the mind into greater peace and alignment with the love of the soul.

When it comes to experiencing an ego death, the mind usually puts up one hell of a fight because it does not want to bend or relinquish the mental conditioning it has learned from a young age in order to feel secure. Ego death is therefore painful for the thinking mind, and while going through it, it is not uncommon for people to experience low mood or depression and struggle with a lack of meaning in life, as well as the sense that they no longer know who they are or how they fit into their old life. Of course, that is the whole purpose of this process. Mental suffering will continue until the mind surrenders to what is and lets go of expectations, faces reality and align with the soul – which is love. Ego death hurts because the old version of a person dies, while a new more compassionate, wiser and soulful version emerges.

Ego death normally occurs in two ways: either with a gradual stripping away of mental activity and long-held ideas that a person slowly recognizes over time are not serving them or, more commonly, as a result of a sudden change in life circumstances that rapidly thrust a person into an awakening. This turbulent change could be instigated by a sudden loss of health, the death of a close relative, a spouse requesting a divorce unexpectedly, or the opposite – falling in love with someone new, outside of an existing relationship, unintentionally. This is what may be referred to in spiritual terminology as a "Tower moment" (taking its description from the Tower card in the tarot deck).

The Tower moment

In tarot, the Tower card represents a sudden unforeseen life event that may look destructive on the surface – bringing a person to their knees initially while circumstances collapse around them – before forcing change for the positive. This could be redundancy from a job, but then setting up a new business venture as a result which goes on to become hugely successful in a way nobody could have foreseen; or it could be the experience of a sudden health scare which leads to living a much healthier and more balanced lifestyle into old age.

When a Tower moment occurs, in the short term there is change that is painful and highly unsettling, but this reveals itself to be wholly beneficial down the line. Tower moments throw a person out of their normal comfort zone and force the mind to recognize it is at the mercy of a power much greater than itself – the soul. The thinking mind is pushed into a realization that it is not in control, and an ego death occurs because those involved have no choice but to turn within and access the deeper dimension of the soul in order to find the strength needed to survive and thrive.

Ego death can occur with any challenging life circumstance, but should ego death occur when a person experiences a deep soul connection while in a loving relationship with another soul, it can be one of the most life-altering experiences a person will ever face. The breakdown of a soul-based relationship feels like total devastation and may affect every aspect of our lives. Physical health becomes disrupted too and it's common for people to experience loss of appetite, inability to sleep, and for old or new health issues to flare up. The mind becomes obsessed and overly focused on the loss of the love, totally distracting the person from being able to cope with everyday life. People often say they struggle to do mundane tasks, like brushing their hair, tidying the house or walking the dog, until they start to heal. A phase of spiritual crisis also often follows, which includes suffering the sensation of core wound pain (which I touched on in Chapter Four), feeling heavy, exhausted and weighed down, plus suffering ascension symptoms (see Chapter Eight).

In order to recover, those who find themselves in Karmic and Catalyst soul connections must learn to see from the soul perspective, take on board the soul lessons being gained, and remember soul love is eternal – even if it is best to physically separate and move on in life from someone for a time in order to find contentment, heal and grow.

So now you've gained greater understanding of the ego death process involved in these soul connections, let's look at their dynamics in greater detail so you can recognize them in your own life.

CALL TO ACTION: Universal intelligence

Learn to see every interaction and conversation you share with another person as the universe communicating to you through them. Everyone is a reflection of a greater intelligence. What is that universal intelligence trying to reveal to you about who you are? Here are two examples to show you how to look for universal intelligence:

1. When someone tells you how much they admire what you are wearing, if instead of feeling self-love you feel self-conscious and play down the compliment, try to see the soul lesson of self-love coming through. At the soul

level this person is reflecting back to you your perfect soul self. Your soul wants you to know you are love. Next time, accept a compliment about your appearance by simply saying "thank you". Remind yourself you are much more than your physical body; you are perfection at the level of the soul and you are loved. Your body is wonderful because your soul chose it.

2. If someone snaps at you for no good reason, stand back. Don't take on their pain. You are indestructible soul energy. No-one else holds power over you. Don't give away your energy to the situation or allow yourself to be sucked in to the drama. If this is a loved one talking to you, you can come back to the conversation when they are feeling calmer too.

Next time someone speaks to you, try to see the soul power that you are reflected back to you by their words or actions. Learn to use every situation and conversation to your benefit. Say this affirmation: "Every experience is a blessing if you use it as a stepping stone."

The Karmic soul connection

When you entered into this physical lifetime, you will have agreed prior to your arrival that certain souls from your wider soul group would cross your path for the purpose of assisting each other on your individual soul journeys. It's important to remember that your soul attracts to you the experiences you need, and not the experiences you want.

The **Karmic soul connection** is the epitome of souls journeying together while helping each other grow. You do this by working through "karmic debt", which is the accrual of ongoing soul lessons yet to be mastered (which may be carried into this lifetime from a prior lifetime). We choose to return with the same soul (or souls) that we began a lesson with in a past lifetime, to learn further from each other this time around. The aim is to tie up loose ends carried over from old storylines, while benefitting from gaining a more all-rounded experience from life.

Karmic connections are usually influenced by conditional love. Those involved in these relationships try to manipulate the connection, holding expectations of what they want or expect from the other person. For this reason, Karmic relationships rarely last. It is likely we will all have several Karmic soul connections play out throughout our lives; Karmic Soulmates can show up in any guise – as a romantic partner, friend, work colleague, mentor or teacher. These souls come and go, creating life alongside you for only a limited time. This means that for as many good times spent together, there will also be drama. The souls involved gradually evolve in consciousness and become soul aware, but that can take many lifetimes. These might be, for example, those who after years of friendship fall out over money and go separate ways, or the live-in lodger/flatmate whose relationship was fantastic at the start but then turns sour resulting in ending the relationship in court. Even some Life Partner soul connections can be Karmic soul connections (more on the Life Partner connection in Chapter Six). The following will help you to identify the Karmic soul connections in your own life.

Signs and indications of a Karmic soul connection

- When you first meet, if the connection is to be romantic, time may seem to stand still as your eyes meet and everything else around you falls away. Your souls recognize each other because you have been together before and there is purpose to your meeting. The universe wants you to know this connection as the important opportunity for further soul growth that it is.

- If the connection is platonic, there will be a sense of immediate connection. You will feel drawn to this person in a way you can't ignore. You like them straight away and eagerly look forward to spending time with them. You know this person has a role to play in your life.
- You enter into the relationship without needing time to get to know the other first because you've met this soul before in another lifetime and you pick up from where you left off. Your soul knows it is eager to get on with the lessons it needs to master and to grow from this connection.
- You soon discover red flags but you ignore them, even though you know in the back of your mind you should not be excusing this person's behaviour.
- You may enjoy talking about this person or showing this person off to friends and family. You will find them attractive because they have something about them you are yet to master. They may be charismatic, beautiful and charming, or be materially successful. Their appearance and what they have attracts you to them. The ego is fed by being with them.
- The relationship becomes turbulent between you. You argue and there's often underlying drama. There are power struggles because the relationship is founded mostly in ego love and therefore control. You love this person but you can't live with this person.

- You hold a fantasy ideal in your head about your relationship and can't see the reality, even when others around you point it out.
- Despite your love for this person, you often don't feel a sense of commitment coming from them. Their actions speak differently to their words. You may walk away because the relationship just doesn't bode well for a long-term happy commitment.
- You may think a lot of this person, but circumstances just don't make it last, e.g. you're not mature enough yet to stay together, career paths diverge, you end up living in different locations, or your connection simply fizzles out.
- When the purpose of your coming together has been served, you both move on in order to attract different soul connections for which your soul is ready.
- After time apart (usually years) and with maturity on your side, you may see what you gained from each other and reconnect, especially if there are still lessons to be gained from each other as part of a Karmic storyline that needs to be completed and released.

All the world is a stage

We've likely all heard the famous quote from Shakespeare's *As You like It*, "All the world's a stage, and all the men and women merely players: they have their exits and their entrances; and one man in his time plays many parts, his acts being seven ages." It's a fantastic literary expression of spiritual wisdom, and describes the role of the Karmic Soulmate perfectly.

Imagine yourself as an actor in the starring role on a stage. You have several co-stars with you in order to create the full storyline, including Soul Family members and Karmic Soulmates.

As part of this, there are actors playing the part of the villains (for every good story must have the element of interest between dark and light). Imagine now that this company of players puts on a show so wonderful that the play is a resounding success. The actors decide to come together again as a company of actors. This time, they put on a new and improved show. They also swap roles, some changing to play the villains with others now taking on the more heroic roles. Once again, the play is a resounding success, but more important than its popularity is that all the actors involved are developing and becoming more experienced, as well as becoming ever more skilled at their craft with every new role they take on.

The role of the Karmic connection in your life is precisely this. Your Karmic soul connections help you to become a fully rounded soul and to come into wholeness within. They help you create the story of your life and, of course, you do the same for them also. Karma should not therefore be seen as something negative, but the opportunity to gain experience from every angle and, in doing so, become ever more skilful at this play we call "life".

DID YOU KNOW? Karma

Many view karma as a type of "debt collection service" in the universe – they make judgements such as, "you were bad to me, so bad things will now come to you" or "you must have lived a bad life before this one in order to experience such suffering this time". In other words, karma equals "you reap what you sow"; but karma is much more complex than this. Other people's actions in relationships cause us suffering with the potential to lift us ever higher into our own soul power. From the soul perspective then, is it possible to judge the actions of another as good or bad at all? In which direction or favour would the soul judge if, ultimately, you have grown ever closer to love because of the difficult situations you've navigated? We can all agree evil exists in the world, but all actions carry both the potential for good and for bad to result from them. Sometimes, really good actions may keep a person comfortable and less motivated to grow and become self-empowered. This may hold a person back from progressing, whereas difficulties propel them forward.

Consider Newton's third law. Sir Isaac Newton stated, "For every action, there is an equal and opposing reaction". When we learn to see that all actions have an equal and opposing force, karma loses its personal vendetta, so to speak. It explains why bad things can still happen to good people, and why bad people often profit in this world – on the face of it anyway. Karma isn't about judgement; it is a universal law. Karma then becomes about learning how to roll with the punches and to use them to transcend.

You can then, more often than not, choose actions that are kind, loving, supportive, uplifting and empowering because it's you who is benefitting the most from taking this action. How others respond to these actions will no longer be of the greatest importance to you. You understand their reaction is their karma. By seeing this, you calm the storm and take the wind out of karma's sails, floating peacefully on calmer waters.

Karmic soul connection purpose

The purpose of the Karmic soul connection is to help you master unconditional love of self and to come into wholeness within by building upon experiences in previous lifetimes along with the soul lessons presented. Once the soul lesson has played out between Karmic Soulmates, these souls naturally gravitate toward other souls with whom they will learn and master other soul lessons, often parting ways with you.

With maturity on your side, and depending on the circumstances, Karmic Soulmates may circle back round in the same lifetime for a further chance to master the soul lessons these unique dynamics present. In time, and with soul love between you, Karmic Soulmates may even become the high vibing Soulmates of future lifetimes.

JAKOB'S STORY

Michael and I hit it off immediately when we met as two married men, away from our wives and young families for the day at a charity corporate event our shared international head office had arranged. We were both in our thirties, and ambitious to better our ourselves professionally and financially. We had a lot in common, especially a shared love of cricket and tennis. We swapped details and stayed in touch, mostly for professional networking reasons at first, but a friendship grew quickly as we began to meet regularly to play tennis together or go to sporting events. Our wives joked we'd formed a bromance. I suppose we did.

I shared with Michael that I was thinking of starting up in business on my own. As a trusted mate now, I asked Mike if I could bounce my ideas off him. I appreciated his knowledge and experience, and I knew he could bring a different skill set to the table because in many ways we were very different characters. What started out as the odd phone call bouncing ideas between the two of us turned into Michael helping me create a business plan, and then from there he and

I discussing going into partnership together. I had the big-picture thinking, but Mike was great at turning that into a practical action plan.

With our wives in agreement, we handed in our notices and went into business. In hindsight, if I had known it would destroy our relationship to do this together, I'd never have agreed to it. Mike and I worked day and night to get our ideas off the ground, and for the first two years it wasn't easy, but we secured several great clients and shared a common vision. At this point, any disagreements Michael and I had were mostly differences of opinion on how to run the business day-to-day, and even though we locked horns from time to time, I just put this down to our commitment to making this work. I ignored the signs that we were actually very different.

We were in the business of providing consulting and training other businesses, and we were doing well for a time for a small set-up before the start of the global pandemic in 2020. As lockdowns were enforced and the country moved to furlough staff, they also adapted their training and consultancy needs. Travel was slashed, our ability to get in front of new clients became near impossible, and people were moved to work from home. Michael and I found our once "sound" business plan no longer working.

As the pressure grew to earn money, the business floundered. This led to frustration and tempers running high. Instead of working together, Mike and I started pulling apart. No-one could have foreseen what would happen down the line, and it became really hard to predict where to focus our energies. We just couldn't seem to agree on the best plan of action. Michael wanted to play safe, but I've always been more of a risk taker and felt we had to be creative. Maybe neither of us were wrong, but it was clear our differing views were becoming insurmountable.

Our relationship became so strained, we barely spoke. Each took responsibility for their side of the business and what was once a relationship based on fun times became the complete opposite. Every phone call between us was pressured, highly strung and frustrating. Then came a major blow as we lost our biggest client. It was a painful time, but I was not ready to cut our loses yet and fold. Mike, on the other hand, without my knowing, applied for a job which he was offered.

I was shocked when he told me he was pulling away. I felt he had let me down by not telling me he wanted out, and I thought he was giving up too soon. He said he was looking out for his family, which I respect, but I was in the same boat and I thought at least we could weather the storm together. We parted ways on really bad terms and I said things I now regret, but these were difficult times emotionally and financially, and Mike was just as cutting. The whole thing was stressful and depressing.

At this time, I came to see Claire for a reading. Sadly, my Nan had passed away a year before, so my wife booked me an appointment. It wasn't something I'd normally do, but having heard my wife's recording of a reading she'd had with Claire, I felt I had nothing to lose. Claire described Nan straight away, and there was no way she could have told me the things she did by researching them. Furthermore, I was surprised when Claire told me I'd started my own business about three years prior and then proceeded to tell me of *my struggles. She even asked me if I knew a Michael, which shocked me. She told me we were Karmic Soulmates, reconnected from a past-life experience in which we were brothers who fought each other, resulting in the death of one of the brothers. We were here to try again. It was a wild idea, but somehow within me it at least now made sense.*

Claire told me there was ego involved on both sides, but we were learning from the other. She felt if we could move past our differences we might be able to reconcile. It was up to us and we had free will. Claire reassured me that my business would be well and that she felt excited about the future. She felt there was an award that would be won. I wasn't convinced at the time as I didn't know if the business was going to be able to stay afloat, but I have since contacted Claire to let her know my Nan was right. My business has stayed afloat despite the anguish, and we just won recognition in a trade magazine. Claire said my Nan felt I had to learn to trust my own inner guidance and instincts and to stand on my own two feet in business. This was the lesson, as well as to work things through with Mike.

I respected Claire's honesty with me in the reading, and it gave me reason to reflect. I have since reached out to Michael because the reading gave me the courage to look at this whole situation from a different angle. We are on speaking terms now at least, and even though I'm still disappointed and I don't think things can be the same, I hope with time we can find the peace I'm sure we both seek inside, because there was a great friendship there originally.

The Catalyst soul connection

The second soul connection in this chapter with the purpose of learning to love yourself as unconditionally as you love others is that of the **Catalyst soul connection**. A much more intense relationship than the Karmic connection, this dynamic is purely soul-based at first, sweeping both people involved off their feet in the euphoria of a universal energy exchange at the heart. This love is soul first and mind second, so is always reciprocated because the soul is love; it can never be one-sided idolization or mental infatuation. The euphoria created, however, inevitably ends when the mind of one or both involved, with all its fears, enters into the fray. When reality strikes in this soul connection, it strikes hard! Neediness, jealousy, addiction, co-dependency – the fall out is devastating as conditions and the need for control drive a wedge between the two. Then one runs, usually without so much as a goodbye, making the pain experienced total.

Catalyst connections are as alluring to the soul as the moth is to the flame. They won't be ignored, even if you understand up front what they are all about. The experience is designed to literally burn your mind, shining a light on all that is wounded and forcing you to focus on self-healing and unconditional love of soul self.

Most people report never having experienced love like it before, and so the memory stays with them for life. Catalyst connections can be so painful that most don't allow themselves to experience love like it again, which is a shame as there is so much to be gained from pure soul love.

For this reason, Catalyst soul connections are usually romantic in nature because the pair get swept up in the energy of pure love and want to merge on every level. That's not to say these connections can't be platonic on occasion (which can be utterly confusing when you fall in love with someone's soul but you are not physically attracted to them). It should also be noted here that it is possible for Twin Flames to act as Catalysts for each other too (see Chapter Seven for more detail on Twin Flames).

The hallmark of the Catalyst connection

Due to the sheer intensity of Catalyst connections, they are usually short-lived, with those involved moving on to enjoy loving relationships within other types of soul connections – such as with Life Partners, who can help support the healing process while they achieve further soul growth.

Catalyst love is Agape pure soul love at the start (see Chapter Two), but the danger is that the parties involved may not be ready to embody such a pure love between them and instead, because fear and ego enter the mix, they close down their hearts. The Catalyst soul connection is the love seen at the start of Hollywood movies, but without the Hollywood happy ending. This relationship goes up like a firework and ends as quickly as it starts. Some Catalyst connections only last weeks, others slightly longer (perhaps a few months to a year depending on those involved), but this connection is classically recognized by its short, sharp, painful nature.

No matter the length of time, the separation is always brutal and painful, triggering a Tower moment. Catalyst connections show us our shadow self, and it may take years following this connection, or even lifetimes, to work through all that is shown in one short relationship.

This soul connection can be seen as a spiritual initiation or "test". Your soul crosses paths with a soul it can so closely resonate with energetically that the power of the pure soul love it creates is experienced as heavenly. Your soul is testing you to see if you're ready to embody that amount of love. You either agree to this type of connection in advance of incarnation, or you may even attract the connection to you organically because you've reached a stage in your own soul awareness where your soul recognizes you are now ready once more for a new level of soul learning. You should congratulate yourself, therefore, if a Catalyst soul crosses your path. Catalyst soul connections usually show up at a time when you're feeling balanced and cruising through life. You may think you've got it all down, then boom! – the energy of this unexpected soul connection knocks you sideways.

The Catalyst soul shows up to take you out of your comfort zone deliberately, and teaches you about yourself in ways you didn't even know you needed. When the Catalyst has fulfilled their purpose, they're usually gone for good, but the inner growth that comes from this experience is eternal. This is a case of "not ready for each other yet"; but who knows, one day, when the time is right, these souls may circle back round each other again – in this life or the next. Alicia's story highlights this perfectly:

ALICIA'S STORY

I met Susanna not long after graduating from university. I decided on a trip away to discover myself before applying for work. I spent treasured time with friends in mainland Europe before heading down to the Mediterranean with a new group of people on the last leg of my tour. It was here I was introduced to Susanna.

We met at a beach party one evening and as soon I saw her, I felt an electric charge go through me, as if something in me recognized her. She pulled up a chair next to me and I could feel her energy before I knew anything about her. It was so strange. I was immediately attracted to this complete stranger who I'd never even spoken to. I couldn't tell if she felt the same, although I noticed she kept looking at me when I turned away. I found it hard to concentrate on anyone else around me. I just had to find a way to talk to Susanna on my own.

I plucked up the courage and casually asked her if she wouldn't mind helping me carry drinks back from the bar to our friends. To my great joy, she agreed and we headed back across the beach together toward the bar area. It was a short walk but it felt like forever because I became so nervous. My heart was pounding out of my chest and then Susanna turned to look at me and said, "I'm sorry, where did we meet before, I can't place it?" As she looked at me, I mumbled, "We haven't met before, but I have the same uncanny feeling." And in that moment, I saw it in her eyes too – something I'd never experienced before, a connection without words. I felt like she looked into my soul. Time stood still.

The rest of the evening was magical. We chatted all night and were thrilled to discover we would be together in the same travelling group for the next month and a half. Over the coming weeks we grew closer still, entering into a whirlwind romance. We just had to be together, so we spent many days on our own, travelling away from the group by day and meeting up with everyone on agreed evenings. Neither of us had felt anything like it – the closeness – before. It was intense. Susanna and I lost ourselves in each other, and these were some of the best days of my life. I never knew love like it. I understand why people say love is a drug. I felt it.

As soon as I got home, I planned to move to where Susanna lived and look for work there. My friends tried to tell me not to jump with both feet, but I ignored their concerns. After all, they couldn't feel what Susanna and I felt. Susanna told me she was on a break from a relationship with a partner she'd been with for five years, hence she went travelling to get some space. She told me that when she got back to the UK, she would give her partner her final answer that they were officially over. She wanted to be with me.

We shared how we felt openly, and I truly believe she, like me, had never experienced anything like this love before. After six weeks of not leaving each other's side, Susanna was the one to board her plane first. The separation I felt at this time was awful. My soul felt like it had left with her. I couldn't eat, I'd lost all interest in travelling and I was miserable company.

On my return to the UK, Susanna and I met up as soon as humanly possible. She told me how much she missed me and that she just needed a few weeks to sort things with her current partner and to be free to move on with me. We stayed in touch constantly at first. She called me telling me she'd told her now ex-partner about me and would be renting a home until they could sell up. We were excited and she invited me up to look at places together as soon as the time was right. As the days went by, however, I noticed Susanna's communications changed in tone. There were no more heart emojis on texts, and I felt her drawing away. She told me she loved me, but I could sense the distance growing between us. I was desperate, so I chased. I invited her to come to see me. I was so relieved when she came and I could feel the connection still so strong between us again. That day we planned when I would be able to see her again, and when she left I felt elated.

Over the next few days I messaged her, telling her how much I missed her already. She answered with merely a heart, which left me anxious again; and then, when I messaged telling her I knew we were meant to be together and I just had to tell her how important she was to me, there was nothing. No response. I panicked. What was wrong? I phoned. No response.

Finally, she called. She told me her ex-partner had begged her to give them another go. She said our love had been too much too soon. I tried to reassure her. I told her it was not a flash in the pan holiday fling. The connection between us was too deep. I demanded love from her and told her I needed her in order to be happy. I left my self-esteem on the floor that day, I admit to myself now. The following day we spoke candidly on the phone, but Susanna told me she could not bring herself to hurt me any more than she was. She said she had deep issues that needed fixing from the past and that I barely knew her. She told me I was manipulating her emotions unfairly too, which shattered me. Back in the real world now, she told me not to contact her again.

The devastation was total. I fell apart. For months I couldn't dress, eat or face life. My parents didn't know what to do with me. They'd never understood me well, but my mum really tried this time and at least this did bring us closer together. Losing Susanna made me question everything: who I was, what I wanted, and why love had not worked out for me. In the end, when I finally accepted Susanna was gone from my life and I needed to move on, I took control. I had to change.

I became resolved to heal myself spiritually and that's when I discovered Claire. Claire's channelling helped me to see what my soul was showing me and I was able to release the pain. I began to see that this experience was not about my being with Susanna in this life, and it never had been. It was about finding myself – the whole reason I went away travelling in the first place. My soul knew exactly what I needed, and I was given the circumstances to help me achieve what I'd asked for. It took time, but I grew in strength and with greater understanding. Now, I can finally say I am grateful for the experience. Susanna and I were not ready to sustain the depth of love we shared, but that is okay. Claire helped me see that the soul bond is there now, no matter what, and I truly hope Susanna is doing well in life. I am happy now and focused on my own well-being. I feel like I can once again take on the world.

CALL TO ACTION: Attachment

Attachment comes from an idea in your head that you could lose something you have, and so you cling on. When we become attached to someone, it is because we have made them part of our own identity. Loved ones become an extension of ourselves. Attachment is a natural emotion which is often confused with love, but the two are not the same. Attachment always causes suffering, because your mind is looking outside of yourself for something you unconsciously believe is missing from you. Look at the list below. Have you ever confused attachment for love? Ask yourself how you might learn to love more and suffer less, by working on releasing attachment.

Attachment	Love
Clinging to someone for fear of missing out on what they are doing, or losing them.	Enjoying the inner knowing that the person you love can go anywhere without you, but the love remains ever present between you.
Longing to see the person you love so much you can't enjoy your time away from them.	You miss the person you love but you are content in the knowing that you'll see them again when the time is right.
Pining after someone when they are not with you. It may feel like a part of you is missing.	Trusting the person you love will come back to you because they enjoy your company, and knowing in the meantime that you are complete on your own.
Avoiding a person because deep down you worry you'll get hurt.	You can explore a love connection because you know you are whole within yourself, no matter what.
Ghosting or ignoring as an attempt to control the other's emotions and how many times this person contacts you.	You communicate openly and express your emotions. You're comfortable to say when you need space.
Stalking social media accounts or looking at photos to see what the person you love is doing because you feel anxious when apart.	You enjoy the time apart because the opportunity to catch up with each other means blissful reconnection. In the meantime, you carry this person in your heart.

Attachment	Love
Feeling jealous of other people spending time with the one you love.	You know you can't be everything to a person. You enjoy knowing other people bring enrichment into the life of your loved one. When they are happy, it makes you happy.
Feeling angry you are not spending enough time with the one you love.	Trusting love shared will always ensure you both create time for each other.
Feeling suffocated. You fear this person will rob you of your freedom.	Secure that love can never smother, but liberates.
Feeling anxious after conversation with the person you love, or worrying that you may have upset them.	You are confident that the love shared means that you are loved for who you are.

Soul addiction

Some soul connections can be highly addictive, leading to obsession and separation anxiety when the two people spend time apart – either temporarily between seeing each other or when the relationship ends for good. Catalyst connections are addictive because the energy of the soul love shared is so intense it leads to a sense of euphoria and feel-good chemicals flood the human body. The connection becomes wholly intoxicating because the amount of source energy created between the two souls is literally breathtaking. This leads to a chemical overload of endorphins that are so addictive – when one of the pair involved in the connection pulls away, the other is literally left with love addiction withdrawal symptoms and must now heal physically, mentally and spiritually. At these times, it is not unusual for people to act totally out of character. They may stalk a person's social media accounts or drive to places where they know the person they love will be (like places of work) just to feel close to them and get a "love fix". They will also want to talk about this person all the time to friends and family, not realizing it's the body's way of boosting feel-good chemicals because of withdrawal.

This behaviour is usually distressing. Those going through love addiction symptoms may be at a total loss to know how to heal within the situation, and find it debilitating until they let go of expectations and see this soul connection for what it is – a stepping stone to a new level of consciousness and a chance for soul ascension. Because of their suffering, they have no choice but to take responsibility for their own mind and heart. Now is the time to focus purely within and to nurture unconditional self-love.

DID YOU KNOW? Love addiction

Love addiction is a real condition. The brain is geared to reward us with feel-good chemicals such as dopamine, oxytocin, vasopressin and serotonin when we experience pleasure. Humans are literally built to seek pleasure, so when a person meets another with whom they fall in love, the body releases these powerful chemicals.

The chemicals usually balance naturally over a period of time and then the pair involved may begin to build a healthy loving relationship. Obsessions can develop, however, when a person becomes addicted to the chemical rush they experience. Chasing the feeling of being "high on love" results in them being overly focused on the person they desire, leading to mood swings, the distortion of reality, emotional dependence, risk taking and loss of control – all signs of addiction and withdrawal. It's important for us all to realize these chemical rushes may be a pleasant side effect that love has on the body, but they are not "love" in themselves and do not last. Research carried out by Rutgers University's Department of Anthropology highlighted that "the reward, addiction and emotion regulation systems in the body are associated mostly with the rejection or loss of love". When love is subsequently rejected or withdrawn, these people suffer with real addiction withdrawal symptoms.

Signs and indications of a Catalyst connection

- This person breezes into your life and turns it immediately upside down. You feel an intensity in the connection you've likely never experienced before due to the purity of the energy created by the two souls merging.
- The connection is soul-based so gender-free. It is more likely to be a romantic connection, although it can also be platonic.
- If it is a romantic connection, the sexual attraction is off the charts because the connection is so deep that the two will want to lose themselves in each other physically as the soul merge takes effect.
- The two souls connect energetically first and you feel a love that is literally out of this world.
- You see in this person what you lack in yourself and you love them for it. They are showing you areas for soul growth.

- This connection happens at any age, to any person. The energy of the love between you sweeps you off your feet – it's not about looks, status, age, race or any earthly concerns.
- Life becomes exciting; you feel you can take on the world.
- You may become addicted to being with this person and love-sick when you are apart. You can't eat, you can't focus, you are addicted to the chemical rush this connection creates.
- Issues not yet dealt with arise from the past suddenly, causing the connection to become toxic.
- The absolute marker of this connection is that it ends abruptly, often with one leaving the other high and dry and even ghosting them.
- A runner/chaser dynamic often plays out, with one person in the connection needing reassurance because of the intensity of the love shared, while the other person fears the intensity of the love and runs away, often blocking contact.
- The heartbreak leads to ego death – you are forced to look at your flaws, insecurities, attachments, fears and co-dependent ways. You see where you need to grow personally and resolve to do better next time.
- You emerge gradually from the experience, changed for good. You are stronger and wiser, more compassionate and soulful.
- You are drawn to a less intense Soulmate connection next time because they offer stability and a chance to work through all you've been shown about yourself.
- These connections are never forgotten, and you may carry a candle for this soul for the rest of your life.

The Catalyst connection purpose

Buckle up if a Catalyst soul crosses your path – you're in for the ride of your life in the relationship stakes, a ride that will force you into greater understanding of unconditional love of self. You are being shown that you're ready to awaken further, and so may be rocketed into the heady heights of divine soul love temporarily. Catalyst connections are never long-lasting because they are so intense, but they leave a lifelong impression. Most of us can't manage the intensity of the energy that this love creates; we certainly don't appreciate the inevitable plummet back towards Earth away from heavenly soul love, along with the free fall that comes with it. This connection leads to a Tower moment in life.

The soul isn't concerned with longevity of a relationship in the physical world. If a Catalyst Soulmate shows up in your life, pay attention. You have been ignoring something that needs healing deep within you and your soul can't move into higher love until you address it. Maybe you don't trust your own resourcefulness enough in life? Maybe you're not living a life with a spiritual outlook just yet? Maybe you give your power away too readily? Maybe you regularly self-sacrifice? Whatever it is, the Catalyst soul connection is here to heal you via tough love. It will demand that these aspects of your personality be acknowledged in order for you to be able to let love heal.

It's normal to see these connections as a curse initially instead of a blessing, but this is to miss the point entirely. Catalyst soul connections lead you back to your soul self, if you let them. What doesn't kill you makes you stronger, as they say, and as an eternal soul you can't die.

Tips for navigating a Karmic or Catalyst soul connection more smoothly

1. Take time in your daily life to reconnect with your soul and bring spiritual practice into your life. Learning to meditate is key. Make your spiritual practice as important as exercise and diet. Develop a new routine. Look after your body, mind and soul as a priority.

2. Recognize the connection for what it is – a wonderful learning opportunity to find self-love within yourself that will lead you back to divine Agape love (as experienced in the spirit world). Remember there are no mistakes. All soul connections have purpose and everything unfolds as it should in order for you both to grow.

3. Address the fear within you. For example, if drama and arguments have become the norm, ask yourself, "What am I afraid of here? Why does this pattern keep repeating? What is this soul trying to show me about myself that needs healing?"

4. Before you jump to judge the other person you are in soul connection with, ask yourself first, "Why I am being triggered by their behaviour? What is it I feel I'm lacking in myself that I need them to give me?"

5. Allow the connection to reveal to you how it will look and what it is you need to learn. Let love lead you; don't try to lead love. The mind cannot control the soul as the soul is the source power from which all else about you is created. Trust in it. It's working for your highest good.

6. Don't ignore red flags. For example, if you feel sad in your soul more than you do happy, if behaviour is abusive, if you are feeling that this relationship is all take and no give,

or if you are always adapting your behaviour around them, these are not healthy dynamics. Have the courage to trust if you need to let this soul connection go for a while; the two of you will reconnect again when the time is right and under fresh circumstances. Soul connections never die, they transform, just like souls. Just because you have met does not mean you should stay together.

7. If you are suffering in the relationship, don't brush it under the carpet and make excuses for this person. Learn to set healthy boundaries and trust in the strength of your eternal soul self.

8. Let go of the need for an outcome in the relationship – for example, in the case of a romantic split, that you need to get back together. Trust in a bigger picture revealing itself to you. The soul will bring you back together when the time is right – in this lifetime or another lifetime. Surrender to your soul journey. You can't always get your own way and nor should you, because we don't always know what's best for us at the level of the mind. The soul knows.

9. Ask yourself before you enter into any conversation or disagreement with the person you are in connection with: "What would pure unconditional soul love do now?" Answer this, and you'll never go wrong.

10. See the term "finding the one" as a term only to be used when discovering your soul self and not another soul. It's not about finding one soul to journey with. It takes many souls to give you life purpose. Learn to love yourself as unconditionally as you do others so you can always be at peace within, no matter what.

KARMIC AND CATALYST SOUL CONNECTIONS

SOUL LESSON FIVE – Painful
Soul Connection Love Heals

We learn just as much from the painful soul connections in our lives as we do those that nurture us. When we think of love, we usually only think of a nurturing experience where we can feel safe and secure just for being who we are.

The spirit guides teach that the soul is always trying to lead us back to the unconditional pure and divine soul love that we are. They teach that until we embody that love consciously, we will attract souls to us that teach us through painful soul connection to find the unconditionally loving nature of the soul within ourselves. We must love ourselves as unconditionally as we learn to love others. This may require a death of the ego and of the way we perceive life, love and the self.

Soul connections are often overwhelming and destructive if approached from the mind and not the heart and soul. Pure love shines a light on all your unconscious weaknesses, insecurities and controlling ways. It highlights fears, and demands you look at your behaviours, handling the negative traits within your personality with a more soulful and loving response. This is the way to free yourself from unnecessary suffering, and the good news is that you are an indestructible soul. You are unstoppable so you can transform your life.

*"There will always be suffering, but one must
not suffer over the suffering."*
Alan Watts

Chapter Six

Life Partners and Soulmates
Soul Connections

"Have you ever met someone for the first time,
but in your heart you feel as if you've met them before?"
JoAnne Kenrick

Everyone wants to find someone in their life with whom they can share a truly loving and lasting relationship. For many of us, that relationship comes in the form of true best friends – the ones who not only get your sense of humour, but are always there for you throughout the years, making you laugh even when things are tough. You know with them you'll never be alone in life, and so we all want to experience the love and joy that comes from a true Soulmate friendship such as this.

We can usually count Soulmate relationships experienced in a lifetime on one hand, but nothing beats journeying with these special souls. Simply put, they get us, without us even having to try. We are loved exactly for who we are, warts and all, and we offer the same honour to them in return. We may not realize it consciously, but when we are with souls such as this, we feel closer to our spiritual home where love abounds and where the soul feels most closely connected to the divine powerful energy source from which it first originated.

A large majority of us also dream of finding such friendship with a romantic partner – someone with whom we can build a home, maybe start a family (including fur family with beloved pets), create financial security, and grow old together. Although it is not necessary for the soul to experience a lifelong romantic pairing in a physical lifetime, it is a natural human instinct to want to share an intimate relationship with another in this way. The Life Partner connection and the Romantic Soulmate connections are wonderful expressions of how the soul manifests within humanity to meet these desires, but with the deeper soul purpose of teaching us how to love another soul unconditionally.

In this chapter, I'll help you to understand more from the soul perspective about both the **Life Partner** soul connection and the **Soulmate** connection (including Romantic Soulmates). In contrast to the Karmic and Catalyst soul connections which teach self-love, these connections are based entirely around the giving of unconditional love to another soul. I will share what I have learned from the spirit guides about these nurturing connections and their deeper soul purpose, as well as highlighting the challenges, as well as the gains, that commonly arise within them. I will guide you to identify these connections in your own life with greater accuracy, as many unknowingly confuse the Life Partner and Romantic Soulmate dynamics. This can lead to unnecessary mental suffering for life partners because people do not yet see their own relationship from the higher soul perspective. By helping you to better understand these wonderfully loving connections, I hope you can navigate your own relationships more smoothly and with greater peace of mind.

Unconditional love feels divine

The purpose of the Life Partner and Soulmate connections is to learn to give pure unconditional love to another soul, freely and completely. In this respect, they demonstrate a polar opposite soul connection purpose to the Karmic and Catalyst soul connections, which are about loving *yourself* as unconditionally as you can love another. Through the giving and receiving of unconditional love, Life Partner and Soulmate connections allow us the secure space that we need in order to grow while navigating the many challenges and opportunities we may face in a physical lifetime outside of the relationship. They encourage us to create adventures and to play too. No relationships in life are ever perfect, because none of us as human beings are perfect. However, these relationships are pretty wonderful on balance. They are so unconditional at times that undoubtedly the biggest challenge a Life Partner or Soulmate connection will ever face is the physical death of their mate. Having spent so long sharing life together, and riding the ups and downs that come with that, losing a mate we love so closely is devastating. Many describe this loss as "soul destroying". I believe this once again to be the unconscious recognition of the trauma felt by the soul, as the subtle energy bodies separate and one soul returns to the spirit world while the other remains in this world.

For the majority in these connections, I observe the paradox to be that it is only when parted by physical death that these souls truly learn the pureness of the unconditional love they shared, as well as its eternal nature. This is because, without worldly material concerns and the ego mind in the way, the pure soul aspect of the love shared now completely shines through. Before this, when both souls were here in this world in human form together, these soul connections tended to require a balance of conditional and unconditional love. Now, because of physical death, the connection moves on to a purely spiritual level. This offers both souls the opportunity to learn that if we can let go of conditions in relationships and love unconditionally in pure freedom, then even in death these soul connections can realize the incredible strength of unconditional pure soul love and its eternal nature.

The Life Partner soul connection

Life Partners and Romantic Soulmates hold similar dynamics as these are the souls who journey with us to help us find security in romantic love, while also providing the opportunity for us to heal wounds from past hurts, both from this life and past lives. While we build earthly lives together, these souls support us in achieving our life purpose here, as we do for them. We become each other's champions, cheering each other along while also navigating the challenges that physical life in this world presents outside of the relationship. In public awareness, the Life Partner connection seems to have been totally eclipsed by the Romantic Soulmate connection, and more recently with the Twin Flame connection (see Chapter Seven). However, based on what I see in my own spiritual practice, the Life Partner connection is likely to be the soul dynamic that a vast majority of us choose to enjoy in life, and I believe it deserves to become as revered as the Romantic Soulmate connection. So many of us have chosen to experience the Life Partner dynamic because of its benefits, yet its steady, reliable and somewhat less attractive image – in comparison to the devoted but enmeshed Romantic Soulmate connection – entices less interest. Nevertheless, it is one of the most emotionally rewarding and balanced dynamics of love possible in the physical world.

The benefit of a Life Partner dynamic

The benefit of the Life Partner dynamic is the emotional and physical space afforded for freedom of inner growth and expression within a long-term supportive relationship. A Life Partner could be a completely new soul connection between two souls who have never journeyed in physical form together before, but find they can share loving harmonic soul resonance. Equally, a Life Partner connection also suits souls who have already journeyed together in previous lifetimes, such as Karmic Soulmates or even Catalysts who have now matured through experience and soul growth while apart and are ready to reunite and journey together once again – only this time to experience a long-term intimate romantic relationship.

Life Partners are commonly the friends who come together as lovers (often much to their surprise) after many years of friendship because circumstances are now just right. They can also be the casual fling that broke up and then picked up again, carrying on to become a more serious relationship – again, much to the surprise of both involved. This is because there is a tying up of shared Karmic soul lessons playing out between them that underpins the relationship. Life Partners grow together in love and respect over time and through each life challenge and milestone conquered together. They look back 20, 30, 40 years later and say, "Wow! Look what we accomplished as a team. Thank you for being there with me through thick and thin."

The hallmark of the Life Partner connection

Life Partners usually experience some form of soul recognition when they initially meet, although it might not be obvious until reflecting back, as they may not consciously recognize the soul bond formed at first. It's not unusual for those in a Life Partner dynamic to experience electrical energy surges within the body upon touching, a sense of immediate chemistry, a deep recognition when looking into each other's eyes, a sense of déjà vu, or dreams of the future together. When this happens, this is because both souls are registering and remembering having been together before in a different lifetime, or having shared time together in the spirit world before they incarnated.

The hallmark of a Life Partner connection, however, is the steady slow growing in love that takes place and deepens over time. This love connection is stable, solid and designed to last a lifetime. In fact, it's common for Life Partners not to really recognize how good they are for each other at the start of their relationship. The beauty of this connection is the depth of their love unfolding over time. Life Partners don't always seem a natural match (even to each other), and when coming together their relationship may be slow or delayed because of this. For example, two people may have known each other for a while, maybe working together as colleagues or as neighbours, before recognizing the strength of the connection or being ready to finally come together romantically. They may also hold completely different interests, have different tastes, and share different views on issues such as politics or spirituality. This means the fit doesn't show itself as obvious straight away, but despite their differences these two still fall in love. Their unique qualities set them up for a wonderful way to learn the benefits of loving someone unconditionally, regardless of differences.

Life Partners find themselves unwilling to leave each other even if things get rough at times. Deep down the soul recognizes that the beauty and purpose of this connection is to stay the course in order to demonstrate unconditional love to another, no matter what.

Signs and indicators of a Life Partner soul connection

- There will be instant physical attraction from the start, but it might not be obvious that this will be a long-term relationship. You commit to each other slowly over time.
- You may get together, break up and get back together again because you do not recognize the connection initially due to a need to experience a Karmic soul connection expression of love first, perhaps. Or, your separation may serve to show you this is a deeper soul love.
- On meeting, you could experience strange energy surges, premonitions, dreams and déjà vu, or deep eye contact that reaches your soul. Your heart may race or skip beats as the soul recognizes and remembers this energetic soul bond.
- You recognize deep within that you are good for one another, even if in personality you may be different, enjoying separate interests and tastes.
- Aside from looks, you may not always understand mentally what it is exactly that attracts you to this person over others. All you know is, you two work and you wouldn't have it any other way.
- This is a real-life relationship with ups and downs aimed to help you navigate the stages of life together. You see your partner's flaws but there's no major red flags.

- This is a well-balanced connection between head and heart, ego and soul. Conditional love plays its part, and the invite is to now love more deeply and unconditionally.
- Insecurities and issues get dealt with through argument or discussion. Either way, you don't walk away. You can't, in fact, even if you reach low points and threaten to. There's a soul agreement here between you that must be seen through and fulfilled. You will not separate until your souls are ready. You are learning the nature of giving unconditional love to one another.
- Life Partners raise children together, co-own pets, create financial security, help each other through health issues, and build a home together. This is practical earthly love. You are here to create a material life together.
- You may not be overly romantic toward each other like Romantic Soulmates often are, and that's perfectly fine with you both.
- These souls usually meet relatively young, from early twenties to early thirties, because raising a family is often part of the agreement. Alternatively, they may meet when much older if another Soulmate connection has been planned as part of a person's soul journey, which happens first.
- Like all soul connections, when the purpose of the relationship has been fulfilled, Life Partners may go separate ways. Love is freedom and not every soul connection stays together in life. However, if Life Partners do divorce after years of marriage for example, these souls remain in each other's lives amicably – usually because there are children involved. Life Partners are around for life. It's Karmic Soulmates that pull apart and separate in painful or hurtful ways.

- Life Partners become part of a person's Soul Family. They may become the Romantic Soulmates of future lives.

Life Partner soul connection purpose

The most wonderful thing about the Life Partner dynamic is its ability to foster independence within the relationship. This is not about becoming enmeshed in each other and living life as one, as Romantic Soulmates do. This is about being loved unconditionally for your differences, while you are also given the freedom to live your life and come into wholeness on your own. The Life Partner relationship lives up to the expression "opposites attract". This love allows the freedom for two seemingly different people to express themselves both within and outside of a romantic partnership, each free to follow passions and dreams away from each other while also being loved by a romantic mate in life.

Because of their differences, Life Partners are not as energetically similar in frequency as Romantic Soulmates. In essence, both are in training, learning that pure unconditional love always requires freedom of expression. For this reason, Life Partner connections are rarely intense loves, but they are usually well-balanced, mostly peaceful and healthy. They allow us to focus on other areas of life that provide valuable soul growth lessons, or for the giving of self to others in service to humanity – something that should be both applauded and aspired to, in my humble opinion. Yet in my practice, I see lots of people complaining about their Life Partners because of the challenges they face due to being so different from one another. Many don't realize their connections are orchestrated to fit the bigger picture of what their soul journey requires, and because of this many don't feel seen or understood. They may mistake the greater freedom their partner allows them in their connection for less love, or they may not feel special enough because they do not see the same gestures being made toward them as they believe they could receive from a doting Romantic Soulmate. This is not true, as Life Partners simply express their unconditional love differently.

It's notable that a Life Partner connection, is an excellent choice of soul dynamic for those souls entering life with a vocation outside of their romantic relationship. The surgeon, athlete, entertainer, entrepreneur, scientist, charity campaigner or politician who wishes to share life with a loving partner but who also needs to dedicate their time to a wider calling or soul purpose in their lifetime does well in a Life Partner dynamic. This is earthly love that works – a balance of learning to give unconditional love within conditioned and conventional settings (i.e. marriage or civil partnerships).

These are wonderful soul connections, and I can't speak highly enough of them because often people can't see what they have "under their nose" if they are busy comparing their relationship to the fantasy ideals seen on TV and film or in music and novels. This connection is about steady soul growth across lifetimes and the opportunity to journey in the physical world, experiencing all its highs and lows, in the company of someone who will provide loving support and security as well as freedom to enjoy creating life within a wider soul group too. Perfection isn't necessary in this relationship, nor is it realistic.

Soul love never dies

I hope you are feeling more confident now, while absorbing the wisdom in this book, to trust that the love you share with others is an energy that exists beyond physical life and death. The physical separation people experience in one lifetime is never the end of a soul connection. Ask anyone who has experienced the death of a close loved one if their relationship ended on the day their cherished loved one died. They will tell you it didn't end, but rather carried on in a different way. We don't forget people just because we become separated in life, or because they die – and we certainly don't stop loving them. Love creates a soul bond that only purifies and deepens during physical separation. This is because the love is no longer tainted by earthly egos and desires. The relationship continues on at the soul level instead, and the task becomes to feel each other's presence existing at the deeper soul dimension.

It is joyful for souls who can resonate in love to journey together. Soul family, Karmic and Catalyst souls, Soulmates, Life Partners and Twin Flames often wait for each other to return to the spirit dimensions before considering reincarnation. From what I see in my interactions with the spirit world, the reunion is worth the wait.

All the soul connections in this book are wonderful examples of love that never dies. It can be mind-blowing to stop for a moment and consider that those you love or have loved deeply in this lifetime have probably journeyed with you before – both in the spirit world and prior lifetimes. Your souls will find each other again one day, and you'll have the chance to express your love completely. I see many people in my private practice that worry or carry guilt around the conditions in which they lost a love. Many worry they were too hard on their loved ones, while others feel they didn't do enough to show those they love how much they care. Is this you? If it is, please know it's natural. It may be time to release the fears and guilt you carry in this way. This is not the end. Those in the spirit world can feel the love you send them. It is comforting when we really grasp that there is an aspect to ourselves that is consciousness, energy, frequency and vibration – eternal by nature. Energy just is and always will be. You cannot die, and nor can your loved ones die. They walk with you still.

DAVID'S STORY

Michelle and I were married for 40 years. I took for granted really what we built together over that time, until one day it was gone. We met while I was in senior year at high school. I felt drawn to Michelle immediately. She was so attractive and, even though she wasn't my usual type, I was drawn to her personality from the start. She held qualities I admired and which I realized I didn't have. That said, we were nothing but acquaintances for quite a few years before we came together as a couple. In our early twenties we found ourselves chatting during the reception dinner at a friend's wedding and discovered we both shared a love of ice hockey. Michelle suggested we attend a game together. A romance grew steadily over time from there.

We were both headstrong and didn't always agree. In fact, many people said we wouldn't last because we were so different in many ways, but something inside me just knew she would be the one I would marry. I remember feeling shockwaves through my body when we first kissed and my heart would race. This is something that was never present when I had dated other women.

Michelle never complained about anything. She ran a hair salon with her sister and was on her feet six days a week until late, but I never heard her complain about it. The only time she took time out was for five years while she stayed home raising our two wonderful sons. She loved her work and was so generous with her time, helping others. She was a workaholic and probably shouldered too much stress, running a small business and a home. I see that now. The only regret I hold now is that we were not afforded more time to enjoy retired life together. I wish it were not this way.

I was devastated the day Michelle collapsed. She suffered a heart attack at home, just before her 65th birthday. To say it was a shock is an understatement. She was full of life and vigour. I could not get over her death. How could she, of all people, have died? She was still young. I was so angry with everything for a long time. We were a team, and living life without her has been too much of an adjustment. We didn't have a perfect relationship by any stretch of the imagination, and I'm afraid now that I may have been too hard on her at times. So, if Michelle sees me writing this, I want to thank her for everything and let her know I love her and look forward to the day we see each other again.

My solace has been in finding Claire and experiencing a reading. It was life-changing for me. Her description of Michelle's passing and her personality was so accurate that there was no doubt in my mind Michelle was communicating *to Claire. When Claire picked up on a specific sign I'd been given, that was when it really hit home that Michelle lives on. Claire told me that I'd heard Michelle calling my name while I was cooking in the kitchen at home since she'd died. I had! I heard her tone of voice so clearly next to me one evening and then smelt her favourite perfume – I was startled. There was no way I should have smelt that scent while cooking food. Claire could only have known this information if Michelle was telling her. I hadn't told anyone. Claire explained that Michelle and I were Life Partners in loving soul connection, and that we had chosen each other in this lifetime and we would choose each other again. She explained our soul journey through this life and helped me see its continuation, even though Michelle and I are now apart. It has given me a sense of peace beyond words to know our love lives on.*

CALL TO ACTION: Sending loving energy to lost loved ones

If you have a loved one now in the spirit world, there may be emotions left unspoken that you wish you'd expressed. Or, you may simply like to continue sending your love to them.

Our spirit loved ones are only ever a thought away. It's never too late to tell them what is in your heart; they receive the energy you send them. You could express your feelings in a love letter to them. You may even receive a sign from them in return, allowing you to trust that they received your love.

- Sit quietly. Focus on your heart and think of your loved one. Feel the love grow between you.

- Write down all the things in a letter that you would like to express but perhaps couldn't say when your loved one was here. You may like to put your finished letter near a photo of your loved one, or place your letter in a controlled and safe fireplace, allowing your words to be carried into the spirit world on the flames.
- It is enough to write the letter and place it somewhere safe. The spirit world doesn't see your words on paper, they feel the emotions you experience as you write the words. Once written, let those intentions go and trust they will be received.
- Don't look for signs. Let your loved one in spirit respond to you in the way they can, *if* they can, and when they can. Maybe they will speak to you in a dream responding to your communication, or maybe a song will play randomly that answers your letter. Perhaps something related to them will appear randomly on your phone or computer. Keep an open mind, and don't dismiss a potential response as simply wishful thinking. If you notice a sign, pay attention to how you feel. Your connection with your loved one is there with you at the level of your soul.

The Soulmate connection

Mostly everyone knows what a Soulmate is, thankfully. Most of us experience the Soulmate connection in our lives. It's not inaccurate to point out that we are all Soulmates to one another because we are connected as "one" at the ultimate level of reality. When I talk of Soulmates here, however, I talk of those with whom we experience incredibly deep bonds of pure soul love. Soulmates resonate so closely, they sometimes can almost read each other's minds. These are the best friends who finish sentences for one another, share passions and interests, and often run projects together. For the same reason, it is not unusual to see Soulmates in business together too.

The reason Soulmate connections are so deeply loving and transformative is that the individuals involved have already released most of the painful karma between them from prior lifetimes. Having ironed out the creases in their soul connection, so to speak, they become free to simply vibe high together without drama getting in the way. Soulmates exist at the same level of soul awareness to one another. It is easy to love a Soulmate with pure soul love, as they see your soul. They love you at the deepest level, beyond even your personality. They know your ego in this lifetime is not the sum total of who you really are, and deep within them, their soul remembers the many lifetimes you've already shared together plus time spent in the spirit world. These are the loves that just get you. A Soulmate can tell you straight to your face when you're out of line and you won't take offence. You know how loved you are by them and you know everything they do and say comes from the heart. If they give you advice, it is in your highest interest to listen. Soulmates recognize there is something special about their bond and even if Soulmates aren't soul aware, they will treasure the specialness of the relationship, because they understand not everybody can share this depth and purity of love with them.

It's important to remember that Soulmates can be platonic and not just romantic, entering our lives as best friends, business partners, teachers, or even pets. (Yes, animals have souls and are conscious sentient beings too.) Soulmates are the family we choose for ourselves. A Soulmate relationship can go wrong if ego is allowed to get in the way of the love shared between them, but usually Soulmates are "ride and die" connections. They journey with you for the duration of your life and orbit round you, both in the physical and the spiritual world. Soulmates choose to journey together over and over again, lifetime after lifetime, because the connection brings so much joy. So, if you have loved and lost a Soulmate in this lifetime, take heart. Your souls will find each other again. The journey continues.

The Romantic Soulmate purpose

Along with the Life Partner dynamic, the Romantic Soulmate connection is one of the most intimate and enduring loves two souls can share. This connection, like the Life Partner, holds the purpose of teaching us the beautiful benefits that come from loving someone else in an unconditional manner. In contrast to the Life Partner connection, however, the manner in which the Romantic Soulmate connection expresses itself is different. Life Partners embrace and love their differences, allowing space for one another to be their own person while loving each other as the two individual souls that they are. Soulmates unite in their similarities; they rejoice in relinquishing individualization and blending together as one. Hence it's the Romantic Soulmates who, upon meeting, will have the instant soul recognition of knowing without a doubt, that they have found "the one".

Life Partners support and encourage one another in their own individuality and celebrate their ability to be separate while also united. Romantic Soulmates on the other hand actually do best when spending most of their time together and blending all aspects of their lives. That's not to say they can't do things apart from one another, they can and do, but these two are happiest when everything they are involved in outside of each other contributes to what they are creating together as one soul team. Romantic Soulmates enmesh in their love – body, mind and soul – and enjoy the experience of living for the other.

Two bookends

I can always tell a Romantic Soulmate connection when I'm working with the spirit world. These two souls are like bookends! One doesn't function well without the other. For example, it's common for people to tell me that within their Romantic Soulmate pairing, they wake up together, eat breakfast together, work in similar industries or share the same interests, raise their kids together, walk the dogs together, eat dinner together and go to bed at the end of the day at the same time together. Eat, sleep, repeat. Romantic Soulmates wouldn't dream of taking a holiday or vacation away from each other through choice – they would simply miss each other too much. They are each other's primary soul playmate in life. If one gets ill, the other often comes down in sympathy. These two are learning about life in unity, so the hallmark of this relationship is that they become like one, even though they are two individual souls. In fact, people almost don't see them as a separate entity after a time. Think of Queen Victoria and Prince Albert as a famous historical Romantic Soulmate pairing, for example.

Romantic Soulmates blend together so beautifully in love that, for all intents and purposes, they soul merge and work toward creating a life that allows them to live as if they are one and the same. They are not the same soul, but they will get as close to being one as they can while living in the physical world together.

When Romantic Soulmates first meet, they recognize the energetic depth of their souls connecting, and even if they are not spiritually minded, they will say things like, "We just knew we were meant to be", "We just clicked", or "As soon as we met we recognized each other instantly". Many report hearing an inner voice telling them, "This is the person you will marry" or saying, "Oh, there you are, I found you again!" Most Romantic

Soulmates see their partner as the most attractive person on the planet, even years later and into old age. Why? Because these are two separate souls, loving each other's soul as one. It was never about their bodies. The purpose of this soul connection is for these two to experience embodying the unity of soul love in the physical world, and to love each other unconditionally as a result.

The challenges of a Romantic Soulmate connection

It's fair to say that society as a whole aspires to the experience of the Romantic Soulmate connection. So many people desire to have one person above all others idolize them – it's the stuff of fairy tales. The reality is that all soul connections are equal, and love should not be judged in hierarchical terms. Soul connections don't work this way. We experience the soul connections most beneficial to us in a lifetime. This takes into account the circumstances of why we incarnated and what we are aiming to achieve as our over-arching life purpose. All soul connections combined work toward the same end: your coming into full soul awareness and unifying with the one divine love of all. Remember, you will be in many soul connections simultaneously in a lifetime. All play a crucial part in reflecting back to you who you really are.

Even Soulmate connections can face challenges at times because no human being is perfect. I have even met several Soulmate pairings who separated for a short period of time, before coming back together again. It happens. However, these souls simply couldn't live without one another. Earlier, I highlighted the merits of the Life Partner dynamic and pointed out that most people overlook them. In reverse fashion, when it comes to Romantic Soulmates, most people overlook the challenges of the connection and focus on the merits instead. I want to highlight to you some of the challenges that the Romantic Soulmate connection faces, in order to provide balance.

Finding "the one"

So many of us are taught to see the Romantic Soulmate connection as "perfection" in romantic love. There is no doubt that Soulmate love is a wonderful experience, even heavenly sometimes. However, all soul connections carry tough soul lessons to master, and I'm sure there will be Romantic Soulmates reading this book who are suffering.

One of the key challenges faced by Romantic Soulmates is that their lives become so blended as one, they unknowingly lose sight of who they are outside of one another. Because they have found "the one", Soulmates readily let their partner complete them, rather than learning to become complete within themselves. This can lead to Romantic Soulmates doing too much for one another in an effort to show how much they love their favourite mate. In daily life, this could be about dealing with something as simple as a dispute with a utility company over an inaccurate bill. You may enjoy being with your Soulmate because they are assertive and a natural leader (maybe they hold a senior position at work). Instead of learning from them and incorporating more of that quality within yourself, you may instead be tempted to let your mate step in to sort out the problems of your own – you allow them to handle the dispute on your behalf. Your Soulmate loves you unconditionally and will willingly take care of tricky problems like this for you, as a show of their feelings. However, allow them to do this too often and you could lose confidence. Your Soulmate could be inadvertently stopping you from learning a valuable soul lesson. Perhaps a way forward would be for them to support you, while you take care of the issue, learning from their advice? Because Soulmates love to do things for each other as an expression of their unconditional love, they often unknowingly encourage each other to fall into their comfort zones. If Soulmates are not self-aware, they can become too co-dependent on one another. Most enjoy the experience of completing each other as it makes them both happy and secure to be this way. What they don't realize, however, is they are unwittingly self-sacrificing for the other. Pure soul love is learning the balance of self-empowerment at the same time as giving love to another, to help them empower themself.

I remember a woman called Maggie coming to see me and becoming frustrated with her husband in the spirit world during a session. Anger is a natural part of the grieving process, and Maggie was angry with him for leaving her too soon because she loved him so much. This manifested in her telling her husband in spirit (while she was with me) that she didn't have anyone now to take her to her dental appointments. She was cross and asked if he understood the difficulties she was facing now that he'd left her behind? She'd become so reliant on her Soulmate to drive her around and generally take care of her, this loss of support following his death compounded her grief. She wasn't coping well without him and so her suffering was made worse. One of the reasons Maggie had loved her husband so much now became a reason for anger and one of her life challenges in learning to journey without him. She'd relied on him totally when he was with her in this life. Maggie didn't have anyone else to turn to. She was now being invited to step into her full power, and achieve things on her own.

Soulmates lead you to find their soul

Over a lifetime, Soulmates are in danger of becoming so totally enmeshed, it becomes impossible to enjoy life without the other. The challenge for the Soulmate remaining in this earthly world after the death of their mate is to learn both the beauty of having experienced loving someone in such depth in this world, and then to use that love as a springboard to open up to the spiritual dimension of life following their mate's death. It will take time, so it's imperative that those who lose a Soulmate take time to heal. The loss of a Soulmate is so painful, it literally feels as if you have lost a part of yourself. It is my experience that Soulmates are regularly driven to the path of spirituality for this reason. They realize now that the love they shared was more than physical, and always soul deep. Given this, they want to know where their Soulmate is. They seek to find their soul.

There is a light at the end of the tunnel and a measure of comfort when the Soulmate "left behind" in this world now learns to find their Soulmate at the soul level instead. This is where their connection has always been and they must discover the truth in this, in order to live in this world without their mate and find a level of contentment. It's important to understand that Soulmates still journey together despite physical separation. Their journey together doesn't end. That journey now takes place between two dimensions simultaneously instead, with one Soulmate taking the spiritual leg of the journey and the other taking the physical leg. It is possible to learn how to remain aware of the connection between you and your Soulmate using techniques such as meditation and after-death communication.

The spirit guides who work with me teach that Romantic Soulmates, separated at a younger age by a premature death in the pairing, already know at the soul level that this experience was part of their agreed Soulmate journey together in this lifetime. The spirit guides lovingly remind both souls that their time will come again one day to be reunited in the spirit world. Until then, they show us that at the spiritual level, the two are never far apart from one another. It's tough soul love, but both Soulmates have no choice but to do the inner work. They journey in parallel between two worlds, working toward finding wholeness within.

Romantic Soulmates who journey through the whole of a physical lifetime together into old age often become the ones who die from a broken heart. It's common for Soulmates who reach an elderly age together to die and return to the spirit world around the same time – even within days or hours or each other sometimes. The blending is so complete with these two souls after so many years of life together, they just don't want to live in the physical world apart. Their soul agreement therefore is managed in a way that they don't have to.

With all soul connections, we must remember there is always purpose to being here together, but also great purpose in being apart. It is possible to love other souls during separation, and there is no reason to feel guilty for this. That is because soul connections express themselves uniquely and do not compete. Love is inclusive. Soul connections of pure unconditional love give us an eternal gift: they open our minds to the soul and to divine love. They remind us of who we really are, even if that remembrance takes lifetimes in this physical world.

LORNA'S STORY

A tall, handsome man named Bill walked in the room and I was transfixed. I felt an instant connection with this stranger that I couldn't explain. It immediately felt right and different to anything else. After weeks of us both creating daft reasons to chat, we got together. We lived in different towns and he was older, but I never doubted for a second that we would last. I knew I would live anywhere in the world with him – and I was not a risk taker! We had a wonderful courtship, and married. Throughout a loving relationship, which had plenty of challenges, we laughed, enjoyed adventures, supported and helped each other. We gave each other confidence and people commented on how right we were together. He was my rock.

Then one evening, he was shouting my name from another room. He had suffered a massive stroke. A huge lifestyle change followed. He was now wheelchair-bound with little speech. After six months of rehab, I became his main carer and we still laughed. Then two years on, another unexpected life-changing stroke. He wasn't expected to live the weekend. Over days, the doctors discussed turning feeding machines off, but I knew Bill was there. Eventually he was heard shouting my name at 3am! Despite being told it never happened in such severe cases, I stood my ground and brought him home five months later.

It was stressful and sad as he was tetraplegic and couldn't speak, but the love never faltered. I loved our quiet times together for that short time. He regained his smile, but a week later his breathing changed. I held his hand, thanked him, told him I loved him and then felt empty. He had gone. I disintegrated. I raged and sobbed. I felt like half of me had been ripped out and taken away. Without him, I had no idea who I was anymore.

Despite warm weather, I felt so ill and huddled under blankets in two of his jumpers. I think that was the start of a spiritual awakening. A message dream from spirit followed and a visitation dream with Bill. That autumn, a mediumship reading provided evidence that Bill was with me. I felt his exasperation at being unable to soothe me. The medium felt intense love.

A series of synchronicities followed which led me to a psychic development circle full of healers, and I could now feel spirit around me. I was to discover who I really was! However, I was still ill with grief and not ready for my new work. At a first reading from Claire, I realized Bill had been showing me signs of his presence for ages: lights flickering, TV turning off; a coffee smell (he loved coffee!).Then one day, I noticed a tilted picture – I knew it wasn't me! I continued in spiritual development, unfolding my latent psychic ability and tried to channel writing with him. That was amazing and still is! Over time I was given the start of jokes where I could only remember the punchline. I got saucy compliments and previously unknown (but verifiable) information about his life before me and the confirmed name of my main healing guide. He asks questions too! Recently, Bill joined my wonderful soul guide reading with Claire and more signs of Bill's love were confirmed. On our twentieth wedding anniversary, I came down to the radio playing and a gold heart on the wall by my seat. He turns lights on in rooms I am entering. He guides me with helpful suggestions, and is so proud of my work. If I am sad, he comes in with love. I feel it in my heart space and that connection is still strong.

Sometimes, I tell him I can't believe we signed up for this soul agreement; that he would go so early. I so miss him here as a human being with me, but do see that my transformation began when he went back to the spirit world. I also see that what he has said is true: "We are still together. Just differently!"

DID YOU KNOW? Country music icons

Country Music icons Johnny Cash and June Carter are a fantastic example of Romantic Soulmates. They were both married to other people when they met. It seems these two both had Karmic Soulmate connections that they would need to work through first, before they could be together romantically in life. June Carter told *Rolling Stone* magazine in 2000. "I never talked about how I fell in love with John. It was not a convenient time for me to fall in love with him, and it wasn't a convenient time for him to fall in love with me. One morning, about four o'clock, I was driving my car just about as fast as I could … I was miserable, and it all came to me: 'I'm falling in love with somebody I have no right to fall in love with.' I thought, 'I can't fall in love with this man, but it's just like a ring of fire.'"

For Johnny Cash, it was love at first sight, and despite feeling the pain of knowing he was in love with June, which would mean they would both suffer painful divorces, the uniting of these two Soulmates would prove inevitable in the end. Their souls couldn't be apart. After prior marriages were dissolved,

Cash proposed on stage to Carter in 1968 and the pair married. Their relationship lasted for the next 35 years, weathering Cash's addictions and health problems and all the challenges that came along with their joint fame. Cash described their love as truly "unconditional" and, in Soulmate fashion, the pair died only four months apart from one another.

Signs and indications of a Soulmate connection

- Soulmates recognize each other straight away at the soul level on first contact because they've journeyed together many times before. There is energetic recognition first.
- Soulmate connections are calm and nurturing. There is hardly any drama between them (despite what might go on in life around them) because they resonate energetically at the soul level so closely.
- There are no major red flags or toxic behaviours toward one another. They've already done all the work in past lifetimes together. This is about bringing unconditional soul love to Earth.
- If it is a Romantic Soulmate pairing, the pair share a sense of "you complete me" and live for one another, doing everything together. They often marry young and have families. Their lives revolve around the little bit of heaven they create between them on Earth.
- Soulmates can become co-dependent and the dynamic can be unhealthy if they aren't consciously aware of the need to create independence between the two of them.
- Soulmates know each other and understand each other so well, it's like they can read each other's minds.

- Soulmates stay in close contact with one another and, if the dynamic is Romantic, this usually extends to public displays of affection such as holding hands and hugging, etc. The outward show of affection in the connection tells the world "You are mine and I am yours". Others often envy this love.
- Soulmates create a safe and supportive environment to heal past wounds. They are safety blankets in the form of another soul.
- The Romantic Soulmate is about finding "the one".
- Soulmates are the "ride and die" connections in life.
- The loss of a Soulmate is totally devastating. The one left behind feels a part of themselves has been wrenched away and is now missing. They are driven to find each other spiritually.

Soul connections work together to raise us higher

Soulmates aren't always meant to be together through the whole of their lives – they are often painfully separated. This is because it is only in physical separation that Soulmates really start to see the eternal nature of the pure soul love they are. What is beautiful, though, is that Romantic Soulmates and Life Partner connections often work in tandem with one another. If it is agreed before birth that both dynamics are to be experienced in the same lifetime, a Life Partner may enter the life of a person after a Romantic Soulmate partnership has ended – or vice versa. The purpose is to help and support the soul left behind in this world.

These soul dynamics are so complimentary, they never compete. Life Partners offer the space needed by the Soulmate, to be able to hold two different deep soul loves in their heart. Similarly, a Romantic Soulmate may enter a person's life after the Life Partner connection ends and do the same, helping to heal heart pain and show a person that love isn't limited to only one soul or soul dynamic.

As I must keep stressing, love is freedom. Love is best shared with many souls and we can never love enough, but as touched on earlier, people often feel guilty at finding love again after the loss of a Life Partner or Romantic Soulmate. Others just feel they couldn't love another because they'd never share the same love. What could top the love they had? I try gently to help these people see that love isn't exclusive – it's inclusive. They don't need to choose one soul connection over the other; they are not betraying their love. Soul connections manifest with their own unique soul purposes and lessons, and the souls involved mostly signed up to experiencing these loves before entering into this physical experience.

As a prime example of how well a Life Partner soul connection and a Romantic Soulmate connection can work so well together in a person's life, I want to share Lissa's story with you here:

LISSA'S STORY

I met my husband, and father of my two wonderful children, late one night on the Northern Line. It was an instant attraction – passing him on the Underground platform in London, I felt a strange rush of warmth. We sat on the tube train, stealing glances and smiles across the carriage when he suddenly got up to leave the train at the stop before mine. I remember my heart lurching in fear that we would lose this moment, but he suddenly mumbled something about having to get off the train and before I knew it, he had somehow reached out a hand which I took, and I jumped off the train with him at Waterloo Station. We stood looking at each other as the tube moved off – two strangers, yet a weird feeling that I knew him somehow. We nervously arranged a date a week later and nearly lost the moment again when we both waited at the same bar, but with me inside and him outside. I waited for an hour thinking that he had stood me up, then finally found him outside. We were like long-lost friends with a remarkable familiarity between us. From that moment we were together for 14 years, built a life together and had two amazing children. Sadly our marriage ended in separation.

After being drawn by my soul to look into past-life regression, I was not surprised to find that he had been my brother in at least one past life. This made so much sense of the dynamic of our relationship in this lifetime on many different levels. I had often felt like he was my brother even before exploring regression. The events shown to me in sessions had a direct link to certain events and dynamics in this lifetime and explained the deep love I felt for him yet also the difficulties in the relationship. There is no doubt in my mind that our soul connection was fated as such. Despite our divorce, I remain grateful to him for so much and am so happy our souls crossed.

Some years later, I attended a Past-Life Regression workshop and I volunteered to be the person regressed at a demonstration. By now, I had trained as a hypnotherapist and wanted to specialize in past-life work myself. While waiting outside the workshop marquee, a man walked toward where I was sitting and stopped, side on, right in front of me. Again, I felt a strong sense of familiarity, to the extent that I even wanted to reach up and touch the tattoo on his arm ... I didn't, of course!

Instead, I entered the tent for the regression demonstration. Unbeknown to me, he came into the tent too and watched me being regressed. He was later to tell me that he felt inexplicably overcome with emotion and had cried watching my regression. We were later put together in a group of other students, and the attraction was clearly a strong one. As we all said goodbye, he and I hugged and it was so strong it was like a physical lightning bolt went through me, I felt like I didn't want to let go of him.

We said our goodbyes and I thought I would never see him again, but by another strange quirk of fate, we reconnected some months later. We were meant to be together and our souls made sure of it. Next year it will be 20 years since we first met. I have done further past-life regressions that have shown me that we have been partners before in several different lifetimes and that this lifetime was our chance to journey together and love each other again. I feel fortunate that our souls were able to find each other. Things haven't always been easy but this is a deep Soulmate connection in which I believe wholeheartedly. I also have no doubt now that I have had previous past-life connections with my children and with other people in my life, and find soul connection an endlessly fascinating and helpful subject.

Tips and suggestions for navigating Life Partner and Soulmate connections

1. Remember to make time for yourself outside of the relationship. When you give so unconditionally to another, you must balance that love with love of self.

2. When your partner pushes your buttons and you argue, recognize they are showing you what still needs healing inside yourself. You do the same for them. Look for the learning for you both – you are wonderful teachers for each other.

3. Your strengths are in your differences and your similarities. Look to see where the other excels and bring more of those qualities into your behaviour.

4. Make time to play. These are high-frequency relationships. Anything that you do together that brings you both joy will naturally elevate your souls.

5. If you are in physical separation currently, try to realize that you are the love you shared. Go into your heart. Feel the love you still carry for your mate. Can you separate yourself from that emotion? No? That is because you and the emotion of love are one and the same thing. If that love is alive in you, it is still alive in your mate. Love is an energy that can't die.

6. Keep an open heart in loving others. If you lose a Life Partner or Soulmate, try to expand the depth of love they showed you out to others who may not have been as fortunate as you in experiencing the love you have shared so soul deeply. Use the lessons you have been shown to unconditionally love others. Resist the urge to cling or claim the love you had as yours exclusively. Use that love

to open the hearts of others. You may just be the teacher another soul was meant to meet on their soul journey toward unconditional love.

7. Try to love in freedom. Recognize that part of sharing pure soul love is learning to let go of trying to control it. If you do, you'll find that love is still there right with you.

8. If your Life Partner or Soulmate is now in the spirit world, live well and live fully, in honour of the love you share. Live the life your loved one can't live with you right now. Create, instead, experiences you can share when you see them again. They're walking with you and they rejoice in your achievements, just as you do with them when hoping that they're doing well in the spirit world. That is unconditional love.

9. Learn to see the wonderful soul lessons that you are being given from this soul connection that cannot die. The journey simply continues in another way.

10. Remember, everything in life has purpose and nothing real is ever lost.

You are already complete

When reading this chapter, it can be easy to feel that you are missing out in life if you have not yet manifested a Life Partner or a Romantic Soulmate connection. In our society, romantic relationships of all kinds are naturally aspired to. Everything we learn and see from childhood sets us up to believe that if we do not achieve a committed long-term romantic relationship in life and build a family together, then we have not succeeded. This is not true. Where does that social conditioning leave those who don't want or can't have children, or those who want to journey alone in life, totally self-reliant? You cannot know the totality of your soul journey here – your soul purpose and the soul agreements that you have made with other souls – until you return to the spirit world. If you do not have a romantic relationship in your life right now, that is perfect. There are lessons and experiences your soul needs outside of a romantic relationship.

When we believe our lives to be incomplete without a Romantic Soulmate we suffer, because we are creating in our mind an idea or fantasy about a love we perceive to be lacking. We imagine we need a relationship in order to feel happy and complete. You are already complete and have always been – love and happiness must come from within first. No-one else can give it to you. They only reflect back to you that which you are.

CALL TO ACTION: Simple breathing

To find peace in your soul relationships, in both the physical and spiritual worlds, try this simple meditation. Maybe you'll feel the love from the guides and your Soul Family in the spirit world coming back to your own heart. You are not alone.

1. Place a hand on your heart, then breathe slowly but deeply. This simple action triggers the body's nervous system to relax. Humans find it comforting as it makes the body feel safe, so it helps to do this in times of grief or stress.
2. As you relax, see if you can still the mind and enter the space of your eternal soul. Think of those in the spirit world that you love. Feel the love you are with them. This will release the endorphins you need to help you find inner peace and heal.
3. Next, send the love that you are outward toward your local area, then out into the country and then out around

the world. Radiate love to those you love in this world and those in the spirit world. Sit in that love and sense the benefit it creates in the body from the peace it brings. Love heals. Now sit in the stillness. Pay quiet attention to all that's around you.

SOUL LESSON SIX –
Unconditional Soul Love Never Dies

The spirit guides demonstrate to us that pure unconditional love is divine. We have the potential to mirror that type of love in our world through Life Partner and Soulmate connections. These soul connections are all about learning to love another soul unconditionally, just as they do in the spirit world.

Everyone in this world desires to find someone in their life with whom they can share a close, loving connection. For many of us, these wonderful soul connections come in the form of Soulmate best friends, Life Partners and Romantic Soulmates. The soul manifests in these dynamics not only to meet our earthly needs and desires, but also to teach us the divine nature of unconditional love. These are the soul connections in which we have the opportunity to gain valuable life lessons while in the security of longstanding nurturing soul connections.

You also learn from the challenges that arise from loving another soul so purely. As wonderful as it is to share your soul journey with your Soulmate best friend, Life Partner or Romantic Soulmate in this life, it becomes incredibly hard to deal with the loss should they return to the spirit world before you. The spirit guides reach out to you now to show and teach you that unconditional soul love never dies. When you lose someone you love deeply due to physical death, it is an invitation for you to find those you love at the level of the soul. When you learn from pain and loss that love only deepens on separation, you also begin to learn the eternal nature of who you truly are. You are the love you give another. They live on in you, and you in them.

"Maybe love at first sight isn't what we think it is.
Maybe it's recognizing a soul we loved in a past life
and falling in love with them again."
Kamand Kojouri

Chapter Seven

Twin Flame Soul Connections

"Love is composed of a single soul inhabiting two bodies."
Aristotle (383–322 BC)

Learning to embody pure soul love and then to share it unconditionally is the main theme running through this book. Love is fundamental to the human experience, but it turns out that the greatest love story in the universe isn't actually between two human beings at all. Rather, it is between the energy exchange of your own soul and a much greater power source than its own, resulting in a divine and blissful union.

Have you heard of a "Twin Flame" or "Twin Soul"? (The terms mean the same.) This idea has become mainstream in recent times, but I had not heard of the term myself until I personally experienced the reality of the **Twin Flame** or **Twin Soul Connection**. Previously, I thought someone's Twin Flame sounded like an endearing expression for a Life Partner or Romantic Soulmate – much like people calling their partner their "other half". I certainly did not know, despite years of working with the spirit world and connecting with souls in the afterlife, that the reality behind these terms (so often innocently referred to erroneously by Romantic Soulmates who think themselves Twin Flames) actually points to a far greater truth about the soul. This truth has absolutely nothing to do with a romantic and intimate partnership at all, so in this chapter I'm going to set the record straight by teaching you the true meaning of the Twin Flame connection and its purpose.

Twin flame connections are not always experienced in every physical lifetime, but because we all have a Twin Soul out there in the universe journeying along in parallel to our own soul, I'm going to help you understand the reality of this connection, as well as share the signs and indications of this sacred soul bond. This is because your path may cross with your own Twin Soul one day (if it hasn't already), and should you meet, you will be seeking all the knowledge you can find about this otherworldly soul connection – as well as guidance on how to navigate the intensity of the soul energy shared between you.

Another reason for wanting to teach you about the Twin Flame connection as we near the end of this book is because, in contrast to Karmic and Catalyst connections that provide soul lessons in loving *yourself* unconditionally, and Life Partners and Soulmates that provide soul lessons in loving *another* unconditionally, the Twin Flame connection is the amalgamation of mastering both these expressions of unconditional pure soul love within a connection that will lead you into direct union with the greatest power source of love there is.

The Twin Flame connection serves the purpose of ensuring that your mind is brought once and for all into alignment with the reality of your own eternal soul, triggering a huge spiritual awakening with the purpose of leading your soul into a state of oneness and harmony with all that exists. For this reason, it is common to meet your Twin Flame later in life, when you have an element of life experience already under your belt. This connection is not about "falling in love" and finding "the one", like Life Partners and Soulmates do; it is the realization *you are one with divine love.* That realization is going to require an elevation in consciousness in the vast majority of us, and the process will likely be as painful and triggering as it is peaceful, blissful and loving.

Busting the myth

Look on the internet and you will see so much romantic fantasy out there. The truth behind the Twin Flame connection has been hijacked and misrepresented, becoming a booming industry on social media, where tarot card readers offer daily predictions on how your own "Twin Flame romantic partner" is feeling, psychic artists will draw your Twin Flame for a fee, and Soulmates living in a happy romantic relationship promise to help you reunite with your Twin Flame when in separation. Popular culture has also painted Twin Flames to be all about painful tragic love, with pop stars and celebrity romances coming under the spotlight. The Twin Flame connection, however, is about something far more important than a physical "love affair to beat all love affairs", and if you try to limit it to such you'll likely not only be sorely disappointed but emotionally wounded too when expectation doesn't match reality. In this chapter, I'll explain the story of your own soul and how it manifests as two spiritual beings, incarnate in two separate human bodies!

Meeting your Twin Flame

When the Twin Flame connection manifests in the physical world, it involves meeting the person who shares the exact same soul energy as you. We all have a Twin Soul counterpart somewhere out there in the cosmos, but whether you cross paths in this lifetime or not will depend on your soul journey and what you came into this physical life to experience.

If you do journey with your Twin Soul in this lifetime, you will meet this person as you might anyone in your life – perhaps introduced to them at work, at an appointment, via email, on social media, when doing the school run or during any normal life activity. However, when you meet, the connection will be anything but normal. A powerful energetic recognition will be unlocked spontaneously by your soul within both of you. It is as though a plug is inserted into its matching power source, bringing the soul completely online and sparking "same soul" recognition and pure soul love. You may or may not consciously notice the energy exchange that occurs initially, but the more you interact in the physical world the more your shared soul energy circuit will build in power and intensity. The result will be that you will not be able to ignore the mental and physical effect this creates. At some point, you are going to recognize that your own soul is reflecting back to you in the form of this other person, and it's going to trigger a huge spiritual awakening in you – and spiritual awakenings don't come easy!

Same soul recognition

In the initial stages of meeting or conversing with your Twin Soul, your mind will register the energetic "sameness" about you both, and the voice in your head might say things along the lines of "I feel I already know exactly who you are" or "I feel like I am with myself when I am with you". Your mind won't be able to grasp what you somehow know deep within you about this person and, if you're anything like me, it will battle to accept that recognition.

Neither of you will mentally understand what is transpiring at this stage as it's nothing you have ever experienced before, but you will know you have never felt such a sense of oneness, total inner peace, pure innocence and pure love within yourself while simply briefly conversing with this person. Your soul is remembering its spiritual "home" and origins, and you will feel a sense of completion within.

In addition, because this is a spiritual connection, it's common for my clients to report such things as spontaneous psychic premonitions, lucid dreams of being with that person that seem absolutely real, out-of-body experiences and astral travel, past-life recollection, telepathy and a whole host of other strange signs and synchronicities that make everyone in the throes of a Twin Soul connection pay attention. Enough to make most of them question their own sanity too!

The challenges arise

Following same soul recognition, the challenges arise. Not only do you have to try to navigate what's unfolding within you in a world that just does not get it while also dealing with a spiritual awakening, but the majority of those I meet also make the obvious mistake of automatically believing that the pure unconditional love being shared indicates the start of an earthly romantic relationship. For example, I met a Twin Soul pairing where one male is heterosexual and the other male is homosexual. The confusion of experiencing pure soul love for each other, despite the clear barrier of differences in sexual orientation, caused distress and upset on top of an already challenging spiritual awakening for the two of them. Each was filled with fear about how to navigate a relationship without being hurt or hurting the other. Until they could be helped to understand the connection, these two struggled with each other and it was painful.

I also know several female Twin Soul pairings who are same sex, heterosexual and married. They were all fearful that the purity of the love between them meant that they had perhaps misunderstood their sexuality, despite being married to Soulmates or Life Partners for years before they met, and not being sexually attracted to one another. For Twin Soul pairings who are sexually attracted to one another, the chances of being physically intimate in these early stages of the connection and then having to suffer the crushing blow of discovering this is NOT going to be a Romantic Soulmate connection is shattering – often leading to devastating break-ups. The two people involved must go their separate ways until time is able to heal the connection and put them on a new footing.

The truth in the connection

If you look at true Twin Flame stories, however, you'll see that the vast majority of people in a Twin Soul connection are not in an intimate romantic physical relationship, and there's no guarantee they ever will be. For good reason too, I believe. This is your own soul conscious energy, manifested within a separate spiritual body and human form. Most of us don't hold a healthy and balanced loving relationship with our own selves, never mind doubling that effect! Your Twin Soul is designed to be the trigger to awaken you to the reality of your eternal soul self and lead you back to divine love. Just by being themselves, they drive you within yourself to heal. As White Feather always teaches, "heaven is a state of being, not a destination".

The Twin Soul connection might not make for a harmonious Romantic Soulmate love affair, but nor will you want it to once you accept what this connection is really showing you about yourself. If you meet your Twin Soul, you will have gained a spiritual partner in crime to help you gain something so desirable you won't even care how the outside expression of your connection has manifested itself in the physical world once you get to grips with it.

Soul healing through the Twin Flame connection

Most people find themselves at a loss to know how to navigate soul-based relationships because they require a level of spiritual self-mastery that we are simply not taught to foster within ourselves. This is why so many Twin Soul pairings end up going their separate ways. They find this intensely energetic soul connection just too difficult to tolerate and balance within themselves. In short, they can't handle the purity of love. This is a shame, and I want to stress it doesn't have to be that way.

Due to the nature of all soul connections, but in particular the intensely powerful Twin Flame connection, White Feather and the team of spirit guides who work alongside him in the spirit world have led my spiritual practice into the field of soul healing and soul connection. They did this in order to help others learn how soul connections work, so people can learn to navigate them successfully, heal and live to their fullest potential, while also finding peace in the understanding that soul love never dies.

White Feather tells me, as humanity evolves in emotional intelligence, more people will experience deep soul connection and be provided with the opportunity to embody soul love on the planet. These connections are incredibly important in making sure we remain connected in a real sense (not just through technology) and that there is harmonious balance between science and spirituality.

Rising above expectations

People usually find their way to me when they are suffering and trying to deal with heartache and confusion. They try to fit soul connection into the ideas they have learned from society about traditional relationships. They hold expectations too, without understanding that soul connection is all about the soul energy dynamics being exchanged and not the ideas being projected by the mind.

For example, a client called Daniel came to me because he had experienced soul recognition in the Twin Soul connection. It happened via a simple social media interaction with Anna, who lived halfway across the world. Due to the strength of the soul energy exchange, Daniel automatically jumped to thinking Anna must be "the one". He told me he had the strongest gut instinct that they were going to be together, and he'd been pursuing the chances of being in a romantic relationship with her. This was causing him much pain because he couldn't understand why, despite the pureness of love shared between them, Anna wasn't responding in the same manner to the connection. I tried to guide my client to see he was missing out on the understanding that the reason he felt they were going to be together was because they were already the same soul energy – it was not because they were a perfect romantic match in the physical world. Firstly, Anna lived halfway across the world and relocation would be a huge issue in itself, but on top of that she was also 20 years older than my client and happily married with a family. Was it really in Daniel's best interests to carve out a romantic relationship with her? His Twin Soul did love him purely, nothing and no one on Earth could affect that, but an earthly relationship in this lifetime would have to take the form of a long-distance friendship. His challenge was to love her in freedom, while realizing the soul bond between them was eternal.

As part of the soul healing, Daniel was also helped by the spirit guides who work with me to see the lessons his soul was teaching him throughout this lifetime's soul journey. He was battling jealousy and possessiveness because he held a fear of losing love, a theme that played out throughout his life, resulting in a number of romantic relationship break-ups. His Twin Soul had shown up to help him heal that pattern, along with other self-reflections that would help him to live a more soulful life. Daniel's Twin Soul was a wonderful gift, but only when he learned to see from the soul perspective, bring spiritual practice into his life and learn to love without expectation and conditions.

The effects of soul recognition and the pureness of the spiritual love experienced in the Twin Soul connection are earth shattering for most. The twins put each other back in touch with the heavenly realms from which their soul belongs, and it becomes highly challenging to ground the experience into everyday life. The experience of same soul recognition shines a light on all the conditional love and fear you've ever experienced in this world, along with the hurt you've acquired, showing you the sheer amount of emotional baggage you still carry as well as the wider issues in this world. The Twin Flame connection forces you to let go of *everything* you've learned about who are, while you remember the eternal nature of the soul and love. Unfortunately, for most people this will lead to a Tower moment, ego death and spiritual rebirth in there lives, that incorporates what they know about themselves now. Which is why, as I said briefly in Chapter Five, the Twin Flame connection can also act as a Catalyst connection.

CALL TO ACTION: Visualization

Your Twin Flame counterpart is out there somewhere in the greater reality. Maybe they are already incarnate in the physical world or perhaps they currently reside in the astral dimensions. If you found your way to this book, you're certainly an awakening soul on the path to greater wisdom, which indicates that you've already come far on your soul journey. The following exercise is designed to help you connect with your soul, while also sending pure love to your counterpart twin.

1. Close your eyes. Now, take three deep breaths and allow the out-breaths to be longer than the in-breaths.
2. Visualize yourself being bathed in pure white light. Feel that light surrounding your body then going into your muscles and every cell, down to every atom, into your energy body while cleansing and healing, rejuvenating and replenishing. Visualize the light settling into your heart and charging your electromagnetic field. See the light cleansing and releasing all past heartache and pain.
3. Now say quietly in your head, "I am love … I am whole … I am soul." Know that where your attention goes, energy flows. Sense the light within balancing your energy and healing your soul. When you feel centred and calm, send love to your twin counterpart too, wherever they are in the cosmos. You two are energetically entangled. You naturally pull each other up in soul awareness and back toward the light of pure divine love. Therefore, wherever they are, wish them well and let them know that you know they are doing their best in life, just as you are doing your best in life.

4. Now, speak kindly to yourself. Take stock. Praise
    yourself for how far you have come on your own soul
    journey. Remind yourself that you have got this. You are
    indestructible and unstoppable. You have lived many lives
    and died many deaths, yet here you are. No matter the
    challenges you face in this lifetime, you can do it. You will
    do it. As you take care of your spiritual and mental well-
    being, you inadvertently take care of your Twin Flame
    counterpart too.

The wake-up call

Most people choose not to talk about their Twin Flame
connection because the experience is so sacred to them and so
paranormal they fear the repercussions of owning the experience
publicly in a world that just won't understand. I myself have felt
the same. However, my life has been dedicated to sharing the
truth about the spiritual dimension of life and the eternal soul.
I only ever teach from first-hand experience, so I find myself in
the position where I feel duty-bound to share a little with you
about my own Twin Flame experience, to help you know I'm
walking the walk while trying to help others struggling to get
to grips with their own soul connections in life. I understand
how isolating the Twin Flame connection can feel, so I hope my
account here helps others.

People cross each other's paths when they are supposed to,
I know that now. There are no coincidences in this life. At the
soul level, a much bigger picture is always playing out. I know
this because, in 2019, I was thrust into the most powerful
spiritual experience I have ever known (and I'd had a fair few
before) when Gyles Whitnall crossed my path and breezed into

my life. Same soul recognition and the Twin Soul connection was instantaneously activated between us. It was an experience completely out of our control, that would rocket us both into expanded soul awareness and which included a shocking "Kundalini awakening" (more on this to follow, but it's enough to say this is a powerful ignition of spiritual energy that physically travels through the human body involuntarily, and leads to spiritual enlightenment.)

Gyles is a fantastic energy healer and spiritual practitioner, but he found his way to me as a regular client. I never know any details about my clients up front (other than their name) due to the nature of my work. However, as soon as we met for his appointment, we were both struck simultaneously by the most uncanny feeling of familiarity about each other. Not in the way you might sometimes recognize a person's face and wonder if you have met them somewhere before – no, this sense of unshakable familiarity was much more intense and accompanied by the most unusual sense of comfortableness together. There was a sense of sameness immediately. It was like we could have pretty much immediately kicked off our shoes, put up our feet, and chilled out with a glass of something cold. Gyles was a complete stranger to me, but I *knew* I knew him already. We would later find out we are complete opposites in ourselves, having led very different lives, and with a large age gap too. Yet when I say I knew him, I mean at the deepest soul level – I knew him as deeply as I know myself! Gyles later told me that, for him, it was like seeing a really close friend again after years of separation and excitedly chatting and catching up with each other on where life had taken us since we'd last met. To me, it felt like I was suffering with a strange amnesia, trying to remember what I knew I should be able to recall. Imagine the mental confusion. The mind was trying to catch up to something the soul already knew, but because we'd never actually met, we still had to go through the usual professional politeness of conversation that two strangers might exchange.

I now know on an energetic level that our subtle energy bodies connected as well upon meeting, when the process of same soul recognition activated. At the time though, I was bewildered. Being highly sensitive, I have often experienced psychic insight when meeting people and coming into contact with their soul energy. For example, when I first began dating my husband, Martin, I saw a clear vision of the two of us living in a house I didn't recognize. Along with it came the wonderful sense Martin and I were now family. Four years later, we would buy the house I saw together, start a family and go on to live a wonderful life together. At the time of the vision, however, it simply acted as a signpost to inform me this relationship with Martin was to be highly significant in my life. I experienced strong premonitions on the birth of my babies too, as well as countless gut instincts and insights over the years about those around me in everyday life.

I have always found psychic ability to be remarkable, and "psychic hits" like the ones mentioned here are always thrilling when they happen – but my encounter with Gyles was in a category of its own. I had never heard of Twin Souls before we met, so after our meeting I simply assumed I'd met a Soul Family member. What we did know instinctively was that something much bigger than the two of us was playing out here. We knew it would involve spiritual growth in some way too, so at the end of that first appointment, when Gyles told me about his interest in energy healing and a desire to develop his mediumship ability alongside this, I offered to help him. We parted ways excited, but neither of us could have even begun to appreciate the enormity of what was unfolding.

Twin Soul activation

It would be a further three months before we met again, and when we did the unusualness of this soul connection truly began to reveal itself. What I didn't know until Gyles and I could feel safe enough together to share our experiences without worrying that we would scare each other away, was that prior to our first meeting Gyles experienced a strange sense of magnetism toward me. He'd discovered my website while searching for a medium and felt a strong pull. However, on discovering my private practice was fully booked for over 18 months, he gave up on the idea of seeing me. However, quite separately to Gyles, his partner Katie was also drawn to me, and sent him a link to my website, which Gyles took to be a sign he should not ignore. During our initial messages about booking an appointment, Gyles began to experience an ever stronger energetic pull toward me. He also reported strange pounding heart palpitations on the day of his appointment that grew in strength as he drove toward our meeting. Strangely though, I too began to experience the same magnetic pull and heart palpitations, coupled with the physical awareness that my heart energy was expanding out as wide as the room around me. I couldn't really detect where it ended, it was so wide. This was heart energy expansion on another level of intensity, triggered by our same soul electromagnetism, and what's incredible is that this symptom stayed at that intensity within me for almost a year!

Over the coming months, we found the bravery to navigate this connection openly together, experiencing the magnetic pull accompanied by the opposite sensation too, a sense that we were repelling the connection (or pulling apart). Although time spent together was always joy-filled, this connection was also hugely intense – sparking ego death, and time spent apart became about the inner self-growth required. This resulted in an energetic and emotionally challenging push/pull effect between us that took a real maturity on both sides and complete trust in one another to navigate. There were many times I panicked that I had scared Gyles away, not just because of the overpowering soul dynamics we were trying to manage between us, but also because of the metaphysical revelations we were gaining, like development of our mediumship and healing abilities, spontaneous psychic insight, telepathy, past-life recollection, Kundalini awakening, states of spiritual bliss and a soul energy exchange that I now know is entirely real. White Feather told us the key to us not repelling one another was to communicate everything between us. That way, we would begin to build trust that what was unfolding at the soul level between us was absolutely real. Communication would help us to observe in real-time the soul effects of this dynamic. The first 18 months were the most challenging. Ego death is painful! All my fears, insecurities and areas for self-growth were painfully highlighted during this time, most of which I didn't even know existed in me, such as a need for control, fear of losing freedom, fear of co-dependency, fear of abandonment, fear of not being good enough, etc. This connection leaves no stone unturned on your path to inner self-liberation and soul freedom. I will say though, the rewards of insight gained are absolutely worth it in the long run.

The spirit guides taught that Gyles and I had come together in this life for a greater purpose. The combination of energy healer and medium in this world joining together allowed us to come under the direct tutoring of the spirit guides, who taught us how to work together as a team. This included learning how to create a combined healing field of energy around our clients that the spirit guides could utilize while Gyles channelled energy healing to the client's own subtle energy body, and I delivered channelled insight from the guides that would support the soul healing taking place in the session.

Twin Soul polarity and parallels

Another mind-bending aspect of the Twin Soul connection is the way Twin Souls mirror each other perfectly. Gyles's and my skills are opposite but totally complementary – as are our personalities. Gyles connects fantastically well with a wide range of personalities and has a way of connecting with someone on a personal level that makes them feel safe to open their heart and heal. I embrace wider audiences through books and public speaking engagements, which encourages people to open their hearts and heal. Gyles is successful in life because he is easy-going and able to go with the flow, while I am the opposite and plan and organize my way to success. At the core, we achieve exactly the same results, but how this manifests in the outer world is always polar opposite. As a surreal upshot of the polarity between us, we observed that our lives seem to manifest in parallel experiences too. For example, we both experienced our spirit guides appearing to us when we were teenagers, lived through parents divorcing, have worked in the field of Human Resources (HR) and recruitment, and we are both spiritual practitioners in our own right. We also both suffered similar health issues around the same time, have family connections with the same town, our grandparents share the same names and our parents the same birth dates. It goes on and on, right down to the everyday level of us both buying or doing the same thing at the same time, independently of each other, in our own individual and separate lives.

It must be stressed that Twin Souls are totally complete and individual in their own right – just like biological twins. You don't lose yourself when you meet your Twin Soul, you gain. We've lost count of the synchronicities between us, and as we watch this unique soul dynamic play out in real-time, we have come to accept that, despite our total independence from each other in our physical lives, at the soul level of reality we are somehow cosmologically entangled. We are one and the same soul force.

Twin Soul Kundalini awakening

The most startling element to a true Twin Soul connection is the spontaneous ignition of Kundalini life force energy that occurs as a direct result of soul recognition. Kundalini is a Sanskrit word meaning "coiled snake", and in Yogic traditions, "Kundalini" refers to a life force energy that sits dormant at the base of the spine until "awakened" (usually through the regular spiritual practice of meditation and yoga exercises). On activation, Kundalini life force energy travels up from the base of the spine to the crown of the head, and it is well documented by yogis that should this "coiled serpent" snake up round the chakras and pour out through the crown, it will accelerate a person's spiritual growth.

Before experiencing it for myself, I didn't believe Kundalini energy was a physical phenomenon; I saw it as a spiritual thing, a concept even, but my goodness how wrong I was! I now know Kundalini energy is a totally unstoppable force of nature once activated. Like water finds the lowest ground, crashing through dams if it needs to, Kundalini energy finds its highest point within the body (the head), seeking out any blockages that need releasing in the subtle energy body on its way up along the spine. In myself, the energy travelled through my physical body and into the field around me in constant waves that felt like they were simultaneously inside my body and in the energy field around me, interrupting my sleep at night and creating such an uncomfortable burning sensation it actually felt like there was a fire physically burning my whole body from the inside out. Because of this, I now believe this energy to be electrical in some way.

The only way through a Kundalini awakening, as far as I can tell, is to patiently wait while your mind catches up with everything it has now been shown and must integrate into your new reality. The mind then quietens down and the energy settles, so you can start to live daily life again as you did before, but from a deeper aspect of your being and with greater spiritual enlightenment.

Validation from the higher realms

Virtually as soon as the connection was established between Gyles and I, White Feather began waking me in the early hours of the morning to communicate directly about the soul, plus the spirit world and soul connection. I shall be forever grateful to this amazing spiritual being who I have grown to trust so completely.

We all have spirit guides walking with us, and they know everything about us. They know our thoughts, our fears and insecurities. White Feather clearly knew mine inside out after a lifetime of union together. So, imagine how absolutely stunned both Gyles and I were when other mediums started receiving communication directly from White Feather. Most of the mediums didn't know me well, if at all, and those who did had no knowledge of my meeting Gyles. Yet still, they contacted me out of the blue, independently of one another. Their overriding message was the same, "Your spirit guide has been to see me with an urgent message for you. He's asking if you understand the importance of who you've just met? Do you understand the connection? It's important you both do, for the sake of your own spiritual growth. You're going to be teaching together as a result of meeting each other, in order to help others."

Of all the messages sent, two spiritual practitioners further validated what I was receiving from White Feather. Firstly, author and angel expert Alexandra Wenman spoke to me during her pre-show chat for an interview on her *Alexandra Wenman Show*. She told me, "your guides have been with me through the night, and again this morning" … and then she reeled off everything that had happened, describing Gyles perfectly and telling me about the past-life visions I'd seen, the purpose of the union and the work we would go on to do together. This was later followed up by a message from aura healer and shamanic practitioner Kathy Mingo, who relayed a similar message, but added, "White Feather wants you to know there will be a soul book as part of this. The two of you will help people understand soul connections, as well as doing joint healing work with your guides. You will also teach. White Feather says the public are now ready to receive deeper truth about the nature of the soul and unconditional love. It's about elevating consciousness in this world."

It's easy to start doubting yourself when going through the Twin Flame connection, but there could be no doubting it now for Gyles and me. Led by White Feather and Gyles's main spirit guide, Juno, we entered a period of intensive spirit-led training that not only developed us as practitioners, but also brought greater spiritual enlightenment to us both.

White Feather teaches on the birth of Twin Souls

I can't write this chapter without sharing the most important teaching that White Feather communicated to me about the birthing of Twin Souls in the universe. He taught me about my own soul's emergence from the light, and encouraged me to be brave enough to share this information with you so others can understand more about their own soul origins too.

I make no claims that the insight received from the spirit world is a scientific account, so please accept this teaching in the way human beings have always traditionally been taught over the course of history – in story form that leads to greater comprehension of a truth that currently lies beyond scientific understanding.

Using the exact terminology White Feather himself used during a channelled session to Gyles and I in June 2021, his teaching is as follows:

"There have been many universes prior to the formation of this one and at the cosmological explosion [the Big Bang] – which was to be the point of inception for this soul's emergence into this universe – the soul seeded as a single ovoid [egg-shaped] conscious light. The light source of pure consciousness originated from the source of all consciousness, which at its core is a great fiery white brilliance, permeating all existence. From this primordial energy light source, the soul passed through a funnel that was dielectric in function and shaped like an hourglass, into the universe. The funnel acted like a cosmic womb, transitioning the soul from its existence in an old universe into the current one we know. During the process

of this incredible cosmological event, the soul ovoid divided into two polarized counterparts. This division is necessary in order for the soul to take form in a universe consisting of dualities. As a consequence, one soul counterpart carries the 'positive' soul energy charge (or what is traditionally known as the divine feminine element) while the other carries the 'negative' charge (divine masculine element). In this way, the two soul aspects become polar opposites, or mirror expressions of each other, reflecting the whole original single soul back to one another."

White Feather described the two counterparts as akin to being the left and right arm of the same body and, aware that he needed to help keep things as simple as possible, he asked us to visualize the yin/yang symbol. The black feminine element of yin and the white masculine element of yang exist as perfectly complete in their own right, but when the two are brought together like puzzle pieces, they reveal that they are indeed a greater unified whole. It's important to remember that the masculine and feminine description here does not imply gender because the soul, being pure energy and consciousness, is gender-free. Instead, "masculine" and "feminine" are words referring to polar opposites. (It may also help to imagine a magnet with both north and south poles.)

White Feather continued by explaining that the soul "twins" could not exist at all if not for the other's existence too and, although complete, perfect and whole as an expression of the soul in their own right, the twins would always be energetically "entangled". I was told that source energy consists of infinite strands of light, each vibrating at its own unique frequency. The twins' united soul originated from a strand of light, unique to that soul. This enables the twins to carry within their soul field a "soul blueprint", or unique soul frequency "hallmark", distinguishing this twin pairing from all other soul twin pairings in the universe and ensuring the cosmic "soul siblings" would ever energetically be able to recognize one another as their counterpart.

White Feather concluded that the soul twins were now free to soul journey throughout reality in parallel to one another. They would gain experience of life in the cosmos, both in physical lifetimes spent apart and physical lifetimes spent together, yet always united within the spiritual dimension of life. Dancing divinely between unity and separation, the twins would act as a unified soul team, gradually working their way to becoming enlightened to their single soul purpose until the time came where they would realize their soul oneness again with pure source energy. You and your own Twin Soul counterpart have truly been heaven sent. Isn't that an awesome insight about your soul self?

DID YOU KNOW? The Big Bang

White Feather spoke in his teachings about a universe before the Big Bang and of a great fiery white brilliance permeating all existence. I find it interesting that physicists themselves theorize there was something before the Big Bang. They now recognize that their understanding of the universe needs to be revisited or expanded upon. They toy with the notion of a model known as an "ekpyrotic" universe – the word "ekpyrotic" derived from the Greek for "conflagration" or "fire", while "pyrotic" means "to burn". So ekpyrotic literally means a universe coming out of the fire.

Physicists also wrestle with the hypothesis that the actual origin of the universe came from a gravitational singularity (which is apparently like a black hole, only monumentally more stupendous). What interests me is that this thinking is not too far flung a notion from the teaching White Feather has given me about the soul travelling through a hyperbola-shaped funnel.

Scientific giant Sir Roger Penrose, who won the Nobel Laureate in Physics in 2020 and who worked alongside Stephen Hawking to develop the "Black Hole Theory", favours the model of a cyclic universe. This would mean the Big Bang would not be the one-off event that began all life, but rather part of an infinite number of bangs and scrunches transitioning one universe into another and creating a cycle of universes. Again this is striking, because it echoes White Feather's teaching that even the infinite soul is subject to a cyclical experience within material universes. Interestingly, Sir Roger Penrose also talks about the mathematics of the Big Bang theory. He teaches that mathematical calculations show that the expansion of the universe begins with photons (pockets of light) and likely ends with photons too, at the collapse of the material universe. I find it fascinating that a renowned physicist talks about the start and end of this current universe as pure light and nothing else. Even if this is just theory, the maths appears to show it's plausible – which excites me based on what I've learned from the spirit world.

FERNE'S STORY

I never believed in Twin Flames or having an "other half". I knew the term was used in soppy novels and films – people finding "the one" and sailing off into the sunset together. My practical nature has always reasoned that there are probably many, many people on this planet that you would be compatible enough to settle down and have a good life with. So, being happily married to a wonderful Life Partner with grown children, meeting my Twin Soul was hands down the LAST thing I ever expected to happen.

He came into my life through my work. A thin, heavily tattooed, somewhat scruffy and depressed young man, 25 years younger than me. Our relationship was strictly professional. My Twin Soul couldn't have been more removed from what I would normally be attracted to in a man. Yet, he felt instantly familiar, and it was obvious that he felt exactly the same about me. I just knew him and we connected immediately. In no time at all, I found myself going from looking forward to seeing him to being utterly overwhelmed by feelings of pure divine love, which then quickly turned into a burning obsession. There was no romance between us at all, but I could not stop thinking about this man.

I knew something was out of the ordinary when my heart burst wide open in a manner I've never known before. I thought about him night and day. His eyes mesmerized me. If I drove past where he lived, I felt a magnetic "pull" toward him, and the closer I got in location the more my heart felt like it would explode. I had sleepless nights, tossing and turning. I didn't need sleep, I was energetically "on fire". I played emotional music that made my heart soar. I awakened sexually, going from not being that bothered to thinking about it constantly. Something had awakened in me and it made NO sense to me at all.

We were from different backgrounds and he was the opposite of me in so many ways. He maddened me sometimes. The puzzling thing was, I KNEW I didn't want to be with him romantically and that it would never work, but I also knew that I loved him wholeheartedly and so unconditionally. It was such a paradox. My heart had been cracked wide open and I felt as if I was going mad. I couldn't tell him. I carried around all this love that didn't have a home. He was drawn to me too, attentive and going out of his way to be with me. We were comfortable with each other, whether chatting amicably or sitting in silence. And the eye contact ... wow. The experience was so intense. On top of this, there was a push/pull dynamic playing out between us. If I pulled back, he pushed to see me more; if he pulled back I felt the urge to be with him, despite the fact I hated feeling this way and fought it with all my being. This connection happened to us and neither of us were in control.

Now, I have fallen in love before but I knew this was something different, as I yearned and longed for him so deeply within my soul that the intensity was painful and inconvenient. I still loved my husband and had no intention of leaving him. This was not about wanting an affair. I was happy with my life: I didn't NEED this!

Fast forward a few years and I am still happily married and my Twin Soul is still around. We meet in a professional but friendly capacity when the need arises. We have never spoken openly about our connection. The purity of love is still there but I feel calmer, and thankfully it does not feel so much of an emotional roller coaster now that I understand better the connection. This has been one of the most challenging experiences I have ever known. I know I was meant to experience meeting my Twin Soul because it has accelerated my own spiritual growth. It has shown me the work I need to do within me. I can be needy and possessive, traits I dislike and didn't even think I had. The soul pull was something

I have never experienced in all my life. This connection will not be ignored once triggered and, one thing is for sure, this journey is not for the faint-hearted!

How do you know if you have met your Twin Flame?

So – the crucial question – how do you know if you've met your Twin Flame? The immediate answer is that if you have to ask if you have met your Twin Flame, then you most likely haven't. Not everyone will in this lifetime, and nor is it necessary. Your mind will always doubt and question when in soul connection with another or when going through a spiritual awakening, but when it comes to the Twin Flame connection your soul just knows.

Most people find their way to Twin Flame information in search of answers, because they are trying to understand mentally what their soul is reflecting back to them. Twin Soul connections are nothing like normal relationships at the beginning and people seek support and help because of them. They often question their sanity.

That's not to say other soul connections can't be intense. Romantic Soulmates or Catalyst connections would think their own connections were overwhelmingly powerful too – love is the greatest power in the universe – but the Twin Flame connection takes intense and powerful to a new level of understanding. I am aware you must experience it to truly know what I mean.

As an example of how unusual meeting your Twin Soul can be, a person who is currently incarnated into this world but who has a Twin Soul that has remained in the spirit world can still experience same soul recognition between them, regardless. If the soul deems that a person's mind is ready for a deep awakening, they will become aware of their twin in the astral dimensions of the spirit world instead. This commonly happens during sleep, and people have reached out to me reporting the symptoms of soul recognition I experienced, but with a soul who isn't even in this world!

It usually starts with a lucid dream, as real as being awake, but the emotional experience that these people are left with afterwards is life-changing. The dreams, although different in storyline, follow a common theme: a being of pure love, who usually refers to themselves as their "divine beloved", meets them and engulfs them in absolute unconditional love. The love reaches them at every fibre of their being, and they know they are loved and accepted in totality – body, mind and soul – no matter their age, health or even poor life choices. The experience is totally healing and transformational. People report these night visitations in their "dreams" lasting all night, and upon waking the love experienced stays with them forever – triggering Twin Soul recognition and activating the metaphysical aspect of the Twin Flame connection in the same way that it affects people who have met their Twin Soul counterpart in the flesh.

One woman, Teresa, reached out to me asking if I could help her connect to her Twin Flame who was resident in the spirit world via a mediumship reading (which I gently declined to do). She told me that she had met her "beloved" several times in the astral dimensions while in an out-of-body experience during sleep. She told me that the experience was spontaneous, she had no control over it and the intimacy shared was like nothing experienced in partnership in this world. In her own words via email, she described the soul merge that took place as an "euphoric crescendo of spiritual energy orgasm, that ended in a divine bursting of my own soul, in pure loving union with my beloved. I then felt oneness with everything and was left in a state of pure bliss upon waking".

She told me she knew from the experience that her Twin Soul no longer needed to be incarnate in the physical world, and was encouraging her now to do her own necessary soul work. The experience it seems was even more incredible than Twin Flames who connect in person. It had triggered the Twin Flame connection within her in a manner that defied belief, and now she was trying to deal with the connection with no prospect of her sharing an earthly relationship of any kind with her Twin Flame in this lifetime. Hence the request for me to connect to the spirit world for her – Teresa was desperate to communicate with her Twin Soul again.

I suggested to her that the point of the encounter was to realize that she is the love of her Twin Flame. It was now about her finding her Twin Flame within her own soul. I suggested she start bringing the practice of meditation into her life and to work on becoming the love she had experienced that night with her Twin Flame. She was bitterly disappointed, but I pointed out that the love she experienced was part of her now. It had been a gift. Maybe she could learn to embody it in this world with a deserving Soulmate just as well. The Twin Soul connection is not about exclusivity, but inclusivity. It's about learning to embody divine soul love for all souls.

Signs and indications of a Twin Flame connection

- Your soul recognizes its soul counterpart instantly upon crossing paths. An energetic soul recognition is triggered at a metaphysical level. Twin Flames don't need to

meet in person to experience soul recognition. Even
a simple email exchange might be enough to activate
soul recognition.

- You feel a strange sense of amnesia, like you are trying
  to recall something about this person that you know you
  should remember.
- You feel a sense of "sameness" or "at oneness" with your
  Twin Flame right from the start. As you connect together
  at the soul level, there is an exchange of pure soul love
  that feels euphoric, but also brings a deep sense of peace
  and completion.
- The connection is spiritual first and foremost; this is not
  about romance.
- Twin souls experience a strong magnetic pull toward one
  another that can't be ignored.
- The connection sparks a huge spiritual awakening and
  rapid soul growth. It is a hugely intense experience,
  especially at the start of the connection. You will be driven
  to become more soulful.
- There is a powerful energy expansion at the heart, creating
  super-strong heart palpitations. The heart is the seat of the
  soul. You feel your heart's energy field expand out into the
  room around you. This commonly brings with it a burning
  sensation in the heart that feels just like a burning flame.
- One twin will be the positive charge of the soul connection
  and the other will be the negative charge of the soul
  connection. This is traditionally called divine feminine and
  divine masculine, but this is not about the gender of the
  two people involved.
- Ego death is a common marker of this connection. It will
  occur as you realize your true soul self and realize the

unconditional love that you belong to in the spirit world. You will let go of a mindset that no longer serves you and it will be painful.

- A push/pull effect plays out as you grapple with the energy of the connection and the dynamics between polar opposite qualities.
- One twin, being the polar opposite to the other, will likely experience intense obsessive thinking that takes up all of their attention (usually the positive charged twin). The other twin will seem to experience the opposite, and doesn't obsess at all. Ego death is occurring no less in both twins.
- One or both twins may try to run away from the connection if they become fearful, or if they feel their twin is trying to control them. They may suddenly cut ties or end the relationship. The experience of separation is devastating because you can't run away from your own soul.
- Kundalini awakening is spontaneously triggered and is a key factor to knowing you've met your Twin Flame. Psychic insights and metaphysical experiences occur (even if you never had a psychic experience prior in your life). For example you may feel as if your twin is physically with you in the room at times, even when they are not. You are feeling them as part of your own soul.
- An inner recognition of being "home" when you are with your twin. Your soul is recognizing its origins from universal source energy and longing to merge with it once again.
- An almost telepathic connection is shared just like biological twins. Twins are completely in tune at the soul level, they read each other's energy without them even speaking. This connection is always soul energy first.

- Because twins are opposites, one twin will often be more readily accepting of the spiritual nature of the connection, while the other turns away from it.
- Perfect mirror dynamic: Twin souls are opposites in personality, yet complement each other. They show each other all their strengths and weaknesses, plus areas for self-growth. They motivate each other to reach for their full potential and to evolve in consciousness.
- During physical separation, "core wound pain" may be physically experienced in the body. Twin Flame separation is painful on all levels.
- There are always huge obstacles in the pathway of Twin Souls, to let them know this is a spiritual connection not an earthly relationship. This commonly includes huge age gaps (the feminine twin is typically much older), marriages, children, living in different parts of the world, differences in religious beliefs, cultural differences and language barriers. Soul love knows no physical boundaries.
- Twin Flames usually meet unexpectedly and later in life – normally after having met Life Partners and Romantic Soulmates. Alternatively, if they meet young, they separate before soul recognition occurs between them. The connection activates later in life when they reunite, years down the line.
- This is *never* unrequited love. Both twins feel the pure love of their own soul energy between them. Love is a given in this connection. A Twin Flame will never intentionally hurt you. Toxic behaviour is <u>never</u> a Twin Flame connection.

DID YOU KNOW? Twin Souls in history

Ancient civilizations passed on teachings in story form. Knowledge of the Twin Soul connection reached us in legend from as far back as the times of ancient Egypt. The Egyptian twin siblings Osiris and Isis were a god and goddess born from Geb (god of the Earth) and Nut (goddess of the sky). They were also married to one another. Note the siblings were twins, being born of gods but married as one. Also note the reference to their being born from the physical (Earth) and heavenly (sky) and the understanding of polarity in this. It seems the knowledge of Twin Souls has existed since time began. Why is this? It's because this is a natural phenomenon, part of the way the universe manifests. "Twin Flame" may be a modern-day term, but the phenomenon itself is timeless.

The push/pull energy dynamics of Twin Flames

A challenging aspect of the Twin Flame connection is the push/pull energy dynamic that plays out between them. Fear is the opposite of love, and when the thinking minds of the two people involved get in the way of the powerfully loving soul energy between them, fear enters the mix and a powerful push/pull effect is created (like an energetic tug of war). Most people in the connection report this as being one of the biggest obstacles they face in the beginning. For example, if one person in the dynamic feels the intensity of pure soul love, but doesn't feel deserving of the unconditional love their Twin Soul reflects back to them, they may try to sabotage the relationship by acting out old behavioural patterns such as accusing their Twin Flame of being over the top with their affections. They then withdraw their own affection, in protection. Their Twin Soul counterpart will feel this pulling away keenly, both emotionally and at the energetic soul level. It's a double whammy and it hurts. They may try to push their twin counterpart to act in a way that makes them feel better, even chasing their counterpart out of panic and desperation. Fear of abandonment is highlighted as an emotional weakness in this other twin now, so the situation arises between them where both twins now have inner work to do on themselves. If that work is extensive, they will most likely part ways until they can reunite and manage the dynamics mentally between them in a balanced and healthy way – without triggering negative personality traits that hurt.

The energy dynamics of the Twin Flame connection is so powerful, should Twin Souls be together in the same room, strangers will even pick up on the energy exchange. Most assume the Twin Flames are together as a romantic couple, but in reality Twin Souls are more like cosmic siblings, even when the connection manifests as a romantic union. Close loved ones often sense the soul purity of the connection between the two involved and because Twin Souls can get along so well, when all is good between them others may try to fit the connection into "normal" relationship templates (romantic or friendship) – and fail. The Twin Soul connection can be perplexing to those around them who don't understand it, as well as to the twins. Many Twin Souls report to me that family and friends actively tried to stop the connection because the connection was so unconventional. What family fail to see, however, is that no one, not even the twins themselves, have power over the workings of the universe and the creation of the soul. An event that happened before the dawn of time is still taking effect between them.

Shadow work and self-transformation

Twin souls are also called "mirror souls". They show you your own soul and mirror back to you absolutely everything that is wonderful about you, but they also highlight everything less than wonderful about you too, including all your insecurities, fears, anger, jealousies, co-dependencies and all your ego's negative traits. Your Twin Flame will highlight the light and the dark within you so clearly because this connection is *all* about self-transformation. If you are needy or possessive, they will be totally freedom loving, highlighting your flaws. Wherever you lack, they will compensate by being the other way, and you do the same for them – vice versa.

The key to the Twin Flame connection becoming a successful union in this lifetime is to become aware within yourself every time you feel triggered and you suffer emotionally over them. Because your Twin Soul loves you purely, they will never hurt you deliberately. So, given this, ask yourself what is it they are mirroring back to you? What is your mind telling you about their behaviour? Are you being realistic? Is it true? Could there be another way to look at things? Remember they are your mirror opposite. Flip the way you look at things on its head to see the truth. When relating with your Twin Flame, ask yourself "What would pure love do now?" This simple question will guide you through the connection and help you to heal your wounds and negative personality traits.

In my own case, for example, I've needed to work hard on letting go of expectation. As someone who loves to set goals and plan, I've had to learn about my need to feel in control. Gyles is a free spirit. I cannot expect him to do what I want when I want, or see things the same way I do. He cannot always be there to work with me on shared work goals and dreams. He has a life of his own, with a partner he loves and family to consider. I can't assert control over him through holding expectations; it would make me feel too sad to treat him like that. Likewise, I'd hate him to assert control over me. I also have a husband I love and a family to consider. I'm a free spirit, too. Therefore, I've learned to let go of all expectation and to trust in both Gyles and the connection. It's liberating! I've learned to let my own soul take the wheel. It's heavenly to know my soul knows my highest good and exactly what I came into this world to achieve, with whom and when. My soul will guide me perfectly – always has – so now I trust in a bigger plan, inclusive of all souls around me.

CALL TO ACTION: Unity with all souls

The Twin Soul connection is about coming into a state of oneness and unity within. Unity is much more powerful than separation, and your soul knows it. It wants you to see both your individuality and your unity with all that is. It's good practice, therefore, whether you have met your Twin Soul in this lifetime or not, to learn to feel a sense of connection to all souls around you and everything. This exercise may help you.

1. Find a time when you can sit without distraction. Take some deep, relaxing breaths and still the mind. Go into your heart and focus on the spaciousness that is your soul.
2. Think of someone that you love. Imagine your soul energy blending with their soul energy in harmony and peace. Now, think of someone else that you love. Do the same, but blend the three of you together.
3. Next, think of someone else and repeat the process. Blending you all together in pure harmony and peace. Repeat as many times as you like. Don't forget the souls in

the animal kingdom too. Feel your sense of inner oneness with everything and the calmness and spaciousness this creates. Liberate your soul. Feel the eternal aspect of your soul being eternally connected to all those souls you love. Sense how connecting with souls you love in this manner improves your physical, mental and spiritual well-being.

4. Extend that blended connectedness out to everything and every soul.

When you change your inner state of awareness, you take the small steps needed for the world to heal and evolve. Repeat the exercise often. Maybe next time, you can think of somebody that you do not love, and include them into the mix, trying to maintain that sense of inner harmony and peace. Learning to look for the soul essence in every living person is an advanced spiritual practice.

Twin Flame separation

As highlighted, Twin Flames usually separate in the early throes of the connection due to the struggle to tolerate the intense energy exchanged. At the same time, they're also famed for coming together and separating over and over again in a lifetime if they can't work through the soul lessons their soul is trying to show them. When the connection doesn't meet mental expectations, wants and ideals, the twins push and pull against each other, arguing, acting out of resentment or jealousy, becoming needy or detaching emotionally in an attempt to control the uncontrollable, or avoiding confrontation. We are all human, after all, but the fall from grace is crushing when we move from the pure love of the soul into conditional love and fear. If the twin pairing cannot see their differences are the very strengths that can lead them to soul union and oneness within, they will most likely require periods of time apart to reflect on behaviour and learn to love both themselves and each other without conditions.

One thing is for sure, Twin Flame separation is painful, and an ego death will need to be triggered in both before they can reunite and come back together in life. It might not feel it, but separation is positive time spent for both to adjust and rebalance the soul energy that they had not yet managed between them. It is also time to reflect, to find self-love, and to heal the wounds being shown as needing attention.

Twin souls are always drawn back to one another. Sometimes it will take time to do the inner work necessary, and people caught up in the Twin Flame connection must learn to be patient and trust in the connection and their own soul. This is a dance that must be done over many lifetimes.

Another reason the dynamics between Twin Flames can be particularly challenging and end in separation is that they are not in conventional relationships. In fact, people find the Twin Soul connection demands non-conformity. That's the point. The soul is pure freedom and for Twin Souls to stay connected to one another in this physical world, they must show love to one another in pure and total freedom. That means: *no expectations, no demands and no needs*. Can you see why these connections are so challenging for people? How many of us are willing to be in a relationship with someone else in this way?

When Twin Flames do separate from one another, it is always because they have soul work to do that requires them to be alone. How long this takes is like asking: "How long is a piece of string?" Perhaps one or both Twin Soul counterparts need to experience other types of soul connections.

If you are in separation with your Twin Flame, don't wait for them in life. You have separated for a reason, and the very act of waiting for them could be holding you back from union. It shows you haven't yet understood that you *are* your Twin Flame, at the level of the soul. Trust that once you've experienced same soul recognition, you two are now on the path to bigger things, either physically in each other's lives or apart.

It's common for Twin Souls who haven't yet come into permanent physical union to move in and out of each other's lives, usually in painful separation. Even when twins are in union (like Gyles and I are), they still have complete and total freedom to move out of each other's lives should they choose. Twin Flames must learn to be as good within their own company and soul as they are when they're in the company of their twin counterpart. This is not a connection of co-dependency, and if you're reading this and longing for your Twin Flame, you have not yet come into completion within yourself. It's a hard truth, but you're not ready to be with your Twin Flame. Each time Twin Flames work on lessons learned and then reconnect they ground more of the pure soul love between them in this world. If you are currently in separation from your Twin Soul, take heart. You will succeed and unite in harmonious union one day if you align with your soul and don't place expectations on the connection.

Meeting your Twin Flame was never really about you being with them physically. All physical life is a temporary experience. This is about realizing the eternal. You *are* your Twin Flame. You are a soul and you are pure love. The connection exists beyond all time. You cannot be separated.

DARSH'S STORY

I dreamed about my Twin Soul before I met her. It was a vivid dream where we were laughing and joking together, and although I didn't know who she was, the love flowing between us was totally blissful and pure. That feeling of love stayed with me for a week, which struck me at the time as highly unusual, but I felt wonderful so didn't really care. Imagine my shock when a few weeks later, I bumped into the very same woman from my dream in real life! I was so confused. I was 55 years old and until that point I had never experienced psychic insight, but there she was in the flesh at an event I attended with work. I recognized her immediately. I felt a strange sense of euphoria deep within and was inexplicably drawn to her. Even more surreal was when a business acquaintance of mine told me he knew her too and I found myself being introduced to her quite naturally.

As soon as our eyes locked, I knew I knew this woman. I didn't know how I recognized her but an unconditional love existed between us. I was at a loss to know how this could this be. Melanie is 15 years younger than me. We are so different to one another – she is vivacious, I am shy; she likes travelling, I like home life; she likes the theatre, I like technology; I have two kids, she doesn't want any – but conversation came easily. The age gap between us was nothing at all. We felt so at home together and, although we were so different, there was a strange recognition of sameness about us. We were both amazed to learn that we had so many similarities in our lives (for example, her dad is a teacher, so was my mother; we both visited Africa in our twenties doing aid work; I'd had knee surgery in my thirties and so had she; we both play the guitar; and, strangely, we share the same birthday).

Melanie's home country is Australia. Just three weeks after our first meeting, she had to return. I let Melanie go without telling her the depth of the love I felt inside, even though I could see in her own eyes she was feeling the connection the same as I was. We continued to speak a few times over the internet, but time zone differences made speaking regularly difficult. Given how well we got along, and despite the distance and differences in our lifestyles, I still began to believe Melanie and I would in some way be together romantically. She was more practical about it, and I began to get frustrated when I couldn't see anything happening. Neither of us could work out what exactly we were to each other and a push/pull dynamic began to play out with intensity. I lived for every message Melanie sent me but, at the same time, I couldn't face the suffering it brought me. I resented being so far away from her, but also didn't want to leave my kids. I was so confused and so totally unprepared when Melanie herself began to avoid talking to me. Things had been great, but she became more and more distant, and the more I reached out to her for reassurance, the worst things became between us. Melanie eventually told me our relationship was too much and she needed space to breathe.

Part of me was relieved, I now knew where things stood, but as we both withdrew, my heart burst wide open and an intense burning feeling made me actually visit the doctor. I never felt so much love mixed with so much pain. I couldn't sleep or eat. Anyone who has not met their Twin Flame is never going to understand that I was soul bereft. I'm a level-headed man in my later years of life. This was not at all what

I expected. I have always walked away from relationships calmly when realizing they were not right. This was not normal to feel like I did and I wanted this whole business gone. I felt I had no power over the love and my world just fell apart. I slipped into depression. Life felt meaningless all because of a relationship that hardly ever was.

It was my mother who suggested I had met my Twin Flame. I admit, I dismissed her at first but in desperation to move on, I researched Twin Flames for myself and that is when I opened up to spirituality. My experience was displaying all the signs of one soul incarnated as two people. I was not of a spiritual mindset at all before meeting my Twin Flame. My old self would not recognize me now. This discovery led to a rapid awakening in a way I would never have expected. I now teach meditation techniques to a small group of people and have taken a great sense of fulfilment from bringing spirituality into my life. I believe my soul was calling to me that night in my dream to awaken for what is to come, and I'm now excited for the future.

Tips and suggestions to help you with a Twin Soul connection

- Remember, the immediate experience of pure soul love with someone you have never met before does not immediately equate to a long-term romantic relationship.
- Although it's much more fun when you are, you don't need to be with your Twin Soul in order to do the inner work. The soul divided into two counterparts and sent you on

your own trajectories in order to gain valuable experience for good reason. This connection is much bigger than this physical lifetime.

- The Twin Soul connection is about your own spiritual awakening. Your soul is trying to wake you up to who you really are. Take up a spiritual practice and learn to get out of the thinking mind and into the spaciousness and freedom of your soul. Listen to music that lifts your spirits, eat well, take care of yourself, do things that make you laugh. Meditate, meditate, meditate!

- Set boundaries. It's okay to tell your Twin Soul if you need space. They are not going anywhere. Even if they run, you will discover your soul in spaciousness. Trust in the connection. If there is space between you, it is in *your* best interest.

- Love yourself. That is what you're being asked to do. Look in the mirror if you have to, and ask yourself "What would love tell me to do now?", especially when you are going through a painful ego death.

- If your Twin Flame triggers you and you feel they are making you suffer because they don't understand you right now, or you think they are treating you in a way that hurts, go within yourself first before you respond. Check for any fears you may be holding. Face the fear first. Then take some space to go back into your soul before you reply. They are your mirror opposite. Flip the way you are looking at things on its head.

- If your Twin Flame is open to and aware of the connection, communicate, communicate, communicate – everything! But only when you are both in a balanced state of mind to do so. This is how you learn to see the reality in the connection.

- Remember ... no expectations ... no needs ... no control. Release attachment to outcome. Love will always do the right thing in a true Twin Flame connection. Fall out of line with love and your Twin Soul will pull away. Remember, love is not attachment – they are two different things. You are repelling your own soul when you come from ego and fear.
- If you are in separation, focus on your goals and dreams and not on your Twin Flame. Do what makes your soul sing. This connection is about you learning to romance the divine from here on in.

The "Twin Flame" purpose and "mission"

Twin Flame connection is about seeing your own soul energy reflected back to you in another person, sparking soul recognition and triggering you into a spiritual awakening. It is a balance between learning unconditional love for self and learning unconditional love for another, which is in fact one and the same thing in the Twin Soul connection – shining a light on a greater truth that we are all love and we are all connected. We are one. Twin Soul connections are therefore about finding oneness within.

To finish this chapter, I'd like to touch briefly upon the topic of sacred union and the "Twin Flame mission", because you may already have heard of this terminology. The term "sacred union" can sound fancy or even religious, but the reason it earns this term with regards to the Twin Flame connection is that the union between yourself and your soul, yourself and your Twin Soul, and your soul and its primordial source energy is truly a sacred expression of how our universe becomes consciously aware of itself. The Twin Flame connection is the story of how souls emerge within the universe and how we are all contributing to a greater universal intelligence. There is no higher mission than that. Therefore, the most sacred union of them all is always going to be between your soul and the primordial energy source from which your soul first emerged. The second most sacred union you will ever enter into is between your self (or thinking mind) and your own soul … and this is where it gets interesting with soul twins.

If the two become soul aware in the same lifetime, and both begin to start living in alignment with their own soul (either together or apart in the physical world), then they are both in sacred union together too. It is then that a really interesting phenomenon can be witnessed: the twins, driven by the same soul energy, may take an interest in the same pursuits despite being polar opposites. Coming from greater soul awareness now, they will become altruistic in their outlook and driven by a higher calling – as all souls do who become spiritually enlightened. (For you do not need to meet your Twin Soul to become spiritually enlightened.) Twin souls in union may find it is now they can come together as a powerful force for good. For example, a Twin Flame pairing that I know personally both work in the music industry. One is a producer, the other a performer. Together they now create music with the aim of awakening the world to greater spiritual truth through sound and song. When Twin Flames are in sacred union, they can achieve wonderful things. This is known as the "Twin Soul Mission".

However, Twin Souls don't have to take on a mission together. There is no failure if they don't, as it may not be the right time. Twin souls separate deliberately in order to have individual experience through many lifetimes. There could be greater gain in spending time apart.

With this in mind, all soul connections have the potential to reach sacred union together. The ultimate goal is to find union with all souls, not just your Twin Flame. Soulmates, Life Partners and Soul Family all have the potential to achieve a state of divine union with you too. Just imagine how heavenly it could be on Earth if we all came together with this level of understanding. It's certainly something to aim for, and the reason I was asked by the spirit guides to write this book.

Signs and indications of sacred union between Twin Souls

- The twins balance the energy of the connection and, despite their polar differences, love each other unconditionally in total freedom, coming back into each other's lives permanently even though they are likely to never form a conventional relationship.
- There is an inner trust shared between the two of "I'm not going anywhere". Neither has to ask the other to stay, and neither are interested in tying the other down. They both understand pure love is freedom, yet Twin Souls in harmonious union find it joyful spending time together, so why wouldn't they do that as often as they can!
- The union becomes sacred and both people involved highly value what they share, even if one twin doesn't yet understand the full spiritual significance of the connection while the other does. Deep down, the connection feels blissful, peaceful and Zen. Like being with yourself.

- There will be a sense of oneness within and an understanding of "I am complete and whole within myself" (in contrast to Romantic Soulmates who feel their partner completes them).
- The twins realize through this connection their oneness with all souls. They move towards unity consciousness, feeling connected to the whole of life.
- The twins' complementary skill sets and interests may motivate them to share a joint vision or goal, known as the Twin Flame mission. Twin Flames pull together while also simultaneously fulfilling their own separate goals and dreams. Freedom is key to Twin Flames. Where Soulmates enjoy being with "the one", Twin Flames seek "oneness within" with the help of one another.

ELIZABETH'S STORY

I met my Twin Flame when I was least expecting it, outside on a cold day at an event at the beginning of 2019. From the moment we spoke, and without knowing anything about her or Twin Flames, I knew without a doubt this was a hugely significant connection and that we had met many lifetimes before. I found her the easiest person I have ever spoken to. (I am married to a man, and my Twin Flame is a woman.)

The connection was so intense that I started to worry about what was going on. In the following months we didn't meet much but there were so many synchronicities, it was mad. For example, songs on my playlist were hugely significant to her, and her birthdate was on the numberplate of my car and also the same number of the building I volunteer in. That number *kept on coming up, and many other things. I knew what she was feeling, and although not a physical relationship, my soul was singing. It was like being in love without the physical contact. The world was a brighter, better place, and I thought about her all the time. We could tell each other everything and felt totally at ease. We are very different: she is a people person, I am not. She is kind, I am learning to be kind. She loves keeping in contact with people, I do not. I love exercise, she hates it. Pretty much opposites, but there was also a complete sameness. It was only a year on I twigged what it was, and I know that on my soul level, she and I are one.*

The relationship fell apart at the beginning of the year. I stepped away as it was too much. We had been arguing for a while because I couldn't accept her views or way of life. I judged and expected. The destruction of a Twin Flame connection is a devastating and hugely terrible event, nothing else matters. I learned that the Twin Flame experience has to be about no strings and no conditions, and I also learned from her a great many other qualities – a better emotional intelligence, to be less judgemental, and so on. It was my decision to step away, and I know it hurt her. Only recently have we spoken over the phone, and I don't know whether we will ever go forward with a better understanding. I do hope so, but it will go as it goes!

SOUL LESSON SEVEN – Twin Flames Reflect the Reality of the Soul

The lesson from the spirit guides in this chapter is that your soul is much more powerful than you thought possible. Your soul energy is manifested in two individual bodies, creating Twin

Souls. Whether your Twin Soul is currently incarnate on Earth, resident in the spirit world, or somewhere else in the cosmos, this divine pairing work together as one soul team. Together they highlight the beauty of being both whole and individual, as well as being "one" with the greater divine universal source energy.

This connection is not for the faint-hearted because it incorporates elements of the soul lessons learned from every other soul connection experienced in your life to date. For this reason, you will likely meet your Twin Flame later in life when you have life experience already under your belt from other soul connections. Having met your Twin Flame, you learn the nature of pure unconditional love in freedom. The spaciousness and inner peaceful state of Zen is the natural state for your soul. In time, as you navigate the Twin Soul connection, you will experience unity together. This will lead you both to see the soul dimension of life reflected back by all souls within your life. You will become totally soul aware.

Your Twin Flame connection may be a hugely challenging experience if you find the spiritual nature of this connection difficult to integrate into your life. It will, however, be the making of you. Your Twin Soul is your living proof of your own eternal soul, the reality of an afterlife, and the existence of universal pure unconditional source love. Could there be a greater gift? This connection is about you learning to romance the divine. Whether your Twin Soul counterpart remains physically in your life or not, their purpose in having entered your life is for you to consciously discover the truth of your own soul's sacred romance with an eternal universal divine source energy ... and *that*, is the greatest love story of them all.

"Ordinary love is selfish, darkly rooted in desires and satisfactions. Divine love is without condition, without boundary, without change. The flux of the human heart is gone forever at the transfixing touch of pure love."
Parmamahansa Yogananda

Chapter Eight

We Are One

*"Souls love. That's what souls do. Egos don't, but souls do.
Become a soul, look around you, and you'll be amazed – all the
beings around you are souls. Be one, see one. When many people
have this heart connection, then we will know that we are all one.
One love. And don't leave out the animals and trees, and clouds,
and galaxies – it's all one. It's one energy."*
Ram Dass

The infinity symbol is a powerful icon representing eternity and the continuation of life and love in a never-ending cycle, echoing the main message of this book. It seems fitting to me, therefore, that this book now naturally finds its way to conclusion in Chapter Eight, as the figure, when transformed 180 degrees to lie on its side, is the infinity symbol.

You and I started our soul journey together in Chapter One, with my explaining to you that you are eternal soul awareness, arising from primordial energy source. Here we are again now, finishing where we began, with the same message – only perhaps this time you receive it with a greater depth of self-realization, which I hope will be of support to you on your soul journey from here.

The reality of life in the physical world is that we love and we lose. When we experience the loss of a loved one, we are driven to find those we are now separated from physically at the level of the soul. My own personal experience of connecting with the spirit world and the souls who dwell there has shown me the existence of a greater reality and total unconditional pure soul love, which is eternal. It highlights to me how little we actually know about life. It has also shown me that humanity and the collective human ego has, in many respects, reached the epitome of narcissism. We are lost in the mind, consciously or subconsciously believing ourselves to be superior to all other life on this planet. The voice in the head and the thinking mind has become so dominant, most of us can barely control it. Yet, many of us now recognize it brings us the greatest suffering.

Fortunately, there is a guiding factor none of us can ignore – the love we experience through soul connection with another. This is a power none of us can control as it happens to us beyond the thinking mind. Pure love is harmony, peace and Zen. It is the unifying powerful force of all life. It is eternal, and it's who you really are at your core.

This is why I am so driven to pass on the teachings from the spirit world. It is also why I have dedicated my life to helping others see from a soul perspective. I see how greater soul awareness heals, how it provides peace of mind, how it unites, how it empowers and informs people's decision making, so they can reach their fullest potential and make the most of why they came into this life. I see how soul healing helps physical, mental and spiritual well-being, and helps us come into harmony within.

Those in the spirit world see this too. They never leave our side, willing us along; and from what they impress upon me, humanity is now at a crossroads, ripe for raising the collective consciousness on the planet. You are part of these exciting times, having signed up for this awesome soul journey. You are on the path to spiritual enlightenment and you will be the real change in this world. Therefore, it's imperative that as many of us as possible come together to live in sacred soul connection.

Heaven sent

You have learned throughout this book that you are on a soul journey of great significance. Your life has great meaning and purpose. You are eternal, and the love you share with others never dies. In Chapter Two, I highlighted that I believe the only question you will ever really be interested in asking yourself when you cross over into the spirit world is, "Did I embody and demonstrate the love that I am well enough and to my fullest capacity?".

I know that you have been drawn to this book because you seek deep within you the understanding of that truth, and to heal through the soul connections that you have experienced in your life. We are all the same. Everyone who comes to see me for soul guidance readings wants to know that their life is on track for fulfilling their soul purpose. They also want to understand that their relationships with those in their lives hold deeper meaning. In addition, they want to know their loved ones in the spirit world walk with them still. They have a need to know they are loved by those they have lost, and that their loved ones in the spirit world also know how much they are loved in return. I wonder if you're the same? If so, this highlights how important love is in your life. It's not just a chemical function of the human body – love transcends this world.

We are all walking around with hurt in our heart caused by experiences with other people in our lives who have, intentionally or unintentionally, caused us grief or pain. Much of that hurt has been caused by our inability to interact with each other in pure soul love. When people come to see Gyles and I for soul healing, and to learn from our understanding of soul connection, it is because they require support in freeing themselves from that hurt and pain, so they can embody unconditional love. They wish to recognize their indestructible soul self too and to discover that it is safe to love in freedom, without fear and condition – healing their heartache and finding peace within. Having learned this, I hope they can now take steps to embrace unconditional love in their lives *before* returning home to the spirit world. Doing so will lead us naturally back to our own soul, where we will always find inner peace, allowing us to experience heaven on Earth.

In order to support *you* in getting there, the theme of this book has been three-fold.

1. Firstly, I have tried to help you understand that you are eternal soul awareness. There is nothing that you cannot weather. You are stronger than you know.
2. Secondly, this book is about your journey toward unconditional love of self. By recognizing that your thoughts create unnecessary suffering and by taking steps to love yourself as unconditionally as you love others, you can make changes in your life for the positive. Learning to see from the soul perspective gives us that clarity. Earth

Family, Karmic and Catalyst soul connections may be painful but they are important because these relationships highlight our inner fears and show us where we must love ourselves more – in order to live fearlessly and to our fullest potential. They help us align with pure soul love.

3. Thirdly, this book is about the nature of giving unconditional pure soul love to others. When you are able to love yourself, and come into wholeness within, you are able to give love to another in a way that will be blissful for you both. Soul family, Life Partners and Soulmates are the loving relationships we experience that help us learn what it takes to love another unconditionally. They also provide security and a safe space in which we can be vulnerable and heal.

All these wonderful soul connections in your life are leading you back to yourself. Then, with greater maturity acquired through many lifetimes of experience, when your soul is ready your Twin Flame can unlock your heart to the purest love you can ever know – universal source love – helping you realize your oneness with all. The highest purpose of your soul is to know itself simultaneously as both individuated from the primordial light source energy from which it emerged, and unified with this powerful universal intelligence. The spirit guides teach we are all working in parallel with our twin counterparts on this return trajectory to unity consciousness and an inevitable soul fusion with a power so great it is beyond our thinking minds and the words in this book. You have been heaven sent on a soul journey to discover that heaven is within you all along – you never really left it.

CALLUM'S STORY

I had always wondered why I had not been able to meet a long-term partner in life. I just never really felt what you hear so many people say about finding a Soulmate, and just knowing they are with the right one. I had enjoyed relationships with a few short-term partners, but these relationships ran out of steam. My last relationship ended badly. There has been nobody who I felt a deep enough connection with that I wanted to commit to for life.

I began thinking there was something wrong with me and was feeling really unhappy. Perhaps I had commitment issues? Perhaps I had spent too much energy on my career? Maybe I should have just settled and given my love to somebody who I wasn't completely in love with? I don't know. I hadn't achieved what so many do: a marriage, a family who can be there for me when I'm old.

When my parents died, I felt the need to seek a deeper truth. I started to explore spirituality, and my path crossed with Claire. Through her work with the spirit guides, she helped me to see that my path in this lifetime had not been about making a commitment to one person. I have always been fiercely independent and my freedom has been my first priority. It probably hasn't helped me at times, but it's who I am, and that's something I am learning to accept. I have a love of animals, and I find it easier to connect with them then I do people. I have realized that I am perfectly well, dedicating my life to my practice as a vet. I have many friends and my life is rich. I always felt like there was something missing within me; I now understand that it was my connection to my own soul that was the missing factor.

Bringing spirituality into my life has helped me to discover that I don't need to be with anyone. The most important relationship I hold is with myself. These days I feel a real sense of deep inner peace and contentment. I have let go of the ideas that were making me feel I had not achieved enough in life. Through Claire's teaching, I have learned that what I am achieving is more than enough. I'm demonstrating love to my friends and to the animals that I help. If I do meet somebody one day, that will be a bonus. It's no longer a source of unhappiness in me. I feel free.

Connection of the bravest

What would the world be like if we could see ourselves as one huge Soul Family on Earth, journeying in freedom and without fear of death? Imagine being able to embrace our differences in the realization that we are learning from each other at the soul level and that all our suffering and pain has great gain. Imagine being able to see that someone is triggering you because you yourself have moved away from alignment with your soul. And imagine recognizing that our differences actually take us closer to the love we are within ourselves, while at the same time benefitting humanity as a whole. How would we adapt the way we relate to others? Would we be more patient? Anger less readily? Be more tolerant and more understanding? Could we find the common ground, where underneath it all we look for the soul within each other – even at times when the people around us are lost in the drama causing harm and destruction? Would we seek compensation and retribution in the same way?

I don't have all the answers, but I do know there will never be peace on Earth while we live in a world where we separate ourselves from each other, without also seeing at the heart of it we are one. Embodying pure love isn't easy, and at times it down right hurts; but we must be brave and, just like the Twin Soul connection perfectly reflects, realize our differences are what can actually lead us to true divine love and heaven within ourselves.

Separation at the physical level from Soulmates, Life Partners, Soul Family and so on becomes an opportunity to reach in deeper and find where the soul connection lies between yourself and those you love. Until you are reunited once again, either in the spiritual world or in this one, those bonds of pure love are eternal. Therefore, we never really can be separated, and we should stop saying that we have lost our loved ones. They are not lost. They are closer than ever. Go into your heart and feel the truth of these words.

We can all learn to consciously interact from a place of higher love within ourselves with every person we are connecting to – even if they themselves are not yet able to interact with us from a place of greater soul awareness. After all, it is easy to love those who resonate closely with us, but not so easy to love those who are your opposite in life, or who simply challenge you – from awkward work colleagues and relatives to grumpy store assistants or dismissive call centre workers. We have to learn how to interact both with ourselves and with others, from a deeper aspect of our being. When you understand that we are interrelated with every soul around us, for better or for worse, you will see that to hurt them intentionally is to hurt yourself with the same force. It works in reverse too, of course.

Ascension symptoms

The levelling up in spiritual awareness that needs to happen on this planet will require that most of us strip away the conditions and the outdated thinking that we inherited from our own childhoods. When you take action to focus on your soul and become more soul aware, your perception on life changes, sometimes dramatically so. You may have taken from this book that life isn't easy for good reason. In fact, the paradox is that the more challenged you are, the more rapidly you will awaken to a higher perspective. The loss of a Life Partner, Soulmate, Twin Flame or Soul Family member can be so devastating, it can cause spiritual trauma, as well as physical and mental illness. It is at these times, however, that we have no choice but to turn within ourselves and find the strength of spirit to survive. We must find the soul bond that exists between us and learn to see ourselves from a soul perspective, while trusting there is a higher purpose.

With a newfound sense of spirituality, you will see changes in your life that reflect your altered sense of self, and they may even seem quite dramatic. Perhaps your whole life circumstances will need to change and you will be required to adapt. Your physical body will likely go through changes too. The mind/body connection is so strong, as your subtle energy body changes, the physical body must then respond too. At this point, it's common for people to report experiencing physical and emotional symptoms that challenge them, such as feeling teary for no reason, developing headaches, and tastes in foods change; they may suffer with insomnia or experience flu-like symptoms. In spiritual terms, these are commonly known as ascension symptoms. I see this levelling up in consciousness almost as a spiritual puberty. Just like teenagers must make the transition from childhood to adulthood and into physical maturity, a spiritual awakening requires you to transition from a spiritually adolescent mindset into a new level of spiritual maturity. This leads to greater wisdom (no matter your age when this happens). You must then learn to assimilate and integrate this deeper level of awareness into your life and to bring it into everyday activities.

Ascension symptoms are a great indication of positive change in your life, so to put you at ease (because they can be troubling) I have listed below the most common ascension symptoms people experience when going through a spiritual awakening. I hope it offers some peace of mind if it is a difficult time.

The caveat to this is if you are currently experiencing physical discomfort or ill health, please don't ignore your physical and mental well-being. If you are suffering and worried, it is best to have a health check with a doctor to rule out something more serious. If you can, try to find someone spiritually minded who you can trust to talk to openly about what you're going through. And, if necessary, seek out the services of a mental health practitioner, spiritual counsellor or spiritual practitioner. It's really hard to go through a spiritual awakening and soul ascension on your own.

Most common ascension symptoms
(this list is not exhaustive)

- Shakes and trembling as more soul energy flows through your being.

- Goosebumps when the mind recognizes soul truth.
- Headaches.
- Loss of sleep. Either you require less sleep due to increased Kundalini energy flow going through your body, or you keep waking up through the night because your brain is hyperactive, processing new understanding.
- Lucid dreams and astral travel when you do sleep.
- Signs and synchronicities (including repeating numbers). You'll notice the universe reflects back to you, like a mirror, everything you're learning about your soul self.
- Flu-like symptoms.
- Flare-ups of old health issues that need clearing and healing.
- Loss of relationships and friendships as you decide to let go of the people who remain in a mindset you no longer resonate with.
- Loss of interest in activities and pastimes you previously enjoyed, and the development of new tastes in music and entertainment, etc.
- Experiencing death of the ego.
- A sense of meaninglessness while you question your life. You are realizing the way you thought about yourself in the past is not serving you – it no longer matches up to who you really are. Nor is reality what you thought either. You don't know who you are now, and that feels uncomfortable to the mind. It does get better over time; this is not the same as depression.
- Tearfulness and feeling overwhelmed, alongside a deeper sense of inner peace.
- Grief, as you mourn the loss of a loved one or your old way of life that you felt comfortable in.
- Becoming more free spirited. The soul is freedom.

- Beginning to dream big, with a want to give back to the world in service. You feel greater empathy and compassion towards people.
- Feeling frustrated with people around you who don't get you. Suffering with loneliness and a sense of isolation until you find new friends with a wider mindset and spiritual outlook.
- Kundalini awakening.
- Daring to make life decisions that are right for your soul. You follow your passion rather than being driven by your head or other people's fears. You start to live fearlessly.
- Feeling the inner calm and strength that comes from emerging into a new and more empowered version of yourself.

Spirit guides and ancestors

This book has been an invitation to see life from the soul perspective, as well as an introduction to understanding the many relationships in our lives from a soul perspective. There are so many unique expressions of soul connections that it is impossible to write about them all within one book. I have had to focus on the most common connections that the spirit world helps me explore in my own spiritual practice, but of course there are many more expressions of soul connection, including the relationships that we hold with the animal kingdom.

We are also in soul connection with our ancestors in the spirit world and our faithful spirit guides and teachers. There are spiritual beings walking with you that you're likely not even aware of, such as ancestors from your family tree going back before you were born. Plus, you are surrounded in love from those in the spirit world who are part of your wider soul group, but who have not entered into this life alongside you on this occasion. So please do try to take heart if you feel lonely in life – be sure to ask for guidance and support from those in the spirit dimensions who walk with you. You are never alone, but you must ask to receive.

In coming to the end of this book, I believe it is fitting to finish with the words of my own spirit guide, White Feather, who has been integral to me being able to bring you the wisdom in this book. I hope the pure love this spirit guide effortlessly radiates toward us all will be felt by you in your own soul. You are loved more than you could ever know.

Communication from White Feather – November 2022

"When you understand that you can never be separated from me, nor any soul from any other, when you come into union with pure love, when you see clearly that you and I are one and the same despite our obvious differences (given that you inhabit a physical body and I do not), when you see that you are never alone and nor could you ever be because you are simply loved too much, that is when you will liberate your soul and enter into an inner state of permanent grace. My heart is your heart, and I will walk with you through a thousand lifetimes, if that's what it takes to bring you into unity with your soul nature and in flow with the great spirit of everything. Little sister, let them know the love of the spirit guides, the higher councils of light and the master teachers is there for all.

We walk with everyone. No soul goes it alone. In your darkest days, we hold a flame to your candle. Tell everyone the news. We can all embody life's greatness. Death is merely a trick of the light. Go forth in our love."

"The soul is an infinite ocean of just beautiful energy and presence made manifest in human form."
Panache Desai

The Violet Flame

Channelled invocation from the spirit guides for healing and transformation using the Violet Flame

The Violet Flame is a wonderfully powerful spiritual energy available to anyone wishing to heal their own soul and transform spiritually. It's suitable for anyone suffering with heartache or wanting to bring healing to their own soul connections. As electromagnetic beings, light permeates our souls. When working with the violet ray of the electromagnetic spectrum, you can release emotional blockages while healing your spiritual body and soul. For this reason, the Violet Flame is the spiritual energy of Twin Flames and all those ready for spiritual healing and advancement. End this book now by sitting quietly, focus your mind and invoke the Violet Flame saying these words, which were given to me from the healing spirit guides who serve alongside me:

I call upon the mighty power of the violet flame now
With palms cupped, I hold the flame here within my hands
I feel it's warmth, I see its colour vivid within my mind
Oh Mighty Violet Flame that spits and flickers
Travel now along my arms and reach my heart
Enter here and radiate through my entire being
Oh Violet Flame, cleanse my weary soul

HEAVEN SENT

Oh Violet Flame, heal my wounds and relieve my heartache
Oh Violet Flame, open my mind so I may see the whole soul
picture before me
Become one with me now
I am the Violet Flame
I am the Violet Flame
I am the Violet Flame
Violet healing rays carry me to my divinity
And here I rest, whole and pure
And here I rest, in loving peace ever more.

Continuing the Dialogue

Now you've found your way to my work, you might like to continue your soul journey with me a while longer. All the services I offer are listed on my website, including how to get in touch with me to learn more about the work that Gyles Whitnall and I do together. Please visit www.clairebroad.com. Be sure to subscribe to my social media also. I have free videos available on my YouTube channel @TogtherwithSpirit, and at the time of writing you can also find me on Instagram @clairebroadmediumship and Rumble @TogetherwithSpirit.

Depending on when you read this book, my work will also evolve with the times, so it's helpful to know I have lots of exciting plans and opportunities coming in the future. My practice is hugely busy, and I find myself in high demand. Availability to see me in person for a one-to-one session may be limited at times. Alongside this, I regularly run workshops and retreats – many with Gyles Whitnall. Together, Gyles and I teach on soul connection and other spiritual topics, including Spirit Release and Soul Healing, plus we offer spirit-led soul-healing sessions. Our work is ever evolving. The aim of all the work I do is to help people become soul aware, heal spiritually and align to a greater love that never dies. If this sounds good to you, I'd love for you to follow my work.

Of course, in the meantime, there's also my two previous books, *Answers From Heaven – Incredible True Stories of Heavenly Encounters and the Afterlife* (which was co-written with *Sunday Times* bestselling author and dream expert, Theresa Cheung) and my own book on mediumship and spirit communication, *What The Dead Are Dying To Teach Us – Lessons from the Afterlife* (which explains spirit communication, mediumship, the afterlife, psychic experiences and the science available in the field of consciousness studies, as well as sharing the true stories of my encounters with the spirit world). Phew! There's certainly lots more for you to explore.

For now though, thank you so much again for giving me your precious time and attention. This book is a deep read, so your being here is not lost on me!

Resources and Further Reading

Key Organisations

Alan Watts Organization (https://alanwatts.org)
Celebrating the life of scholar and philosopher Alan Watts.

HeartMath Institute (www.heartmath.org)
Since 1991, the HeartMath Institute has developed reliable, scientifically validated tools that help people reduce and avoid stress while experiencing increased peace, satisfaction and self-security. Research at the HeartMath Institute shows that adding heart to our daily activities and connections produces measurable benefits to our own and others' well-being.

Krishnamurti Foundation (www.jkrishnamurti.org)
J. Krishnamurti Online is a unique initiative of the four Krishnamurti Foundations to make the teachings of philosopher J. Krishnamurti freely available, downloadable and to guarantee authenticity.

Love Serve Remember Foundation (www.ramdass.org)
Dedicated to preserving and continuing the teachings of guru Neem Karoli Baba and psychologist and psychedelic pioneer Ram Dass.

Sri Ramana Maharshi (www.sriramanamaharshi.org)

The College of Psychic Studies (www.collegeofpsychicstudies. co.uk)
Founded in 1884 by a group of eminent scholars and scientists, the College of Psychic Studies is based in Kensington, London and runs cutting-edge courses in psychic development where modern methods are used.

The Institute of Noetic Sciences (IONS) (www.noetic.org)
Science-based, non-profit research, education and membership organization dedicated to consciousness research and educational

outreach, and engaging a global learning community in the realization of human potential.

The Institute of Spiritualist Mediums (www.ism.org.uk)
Charitable organization set-up for the promotion, teaching and development of spirit communication.

The Society for Psychical Research (www.spr.ac.uk)
Founded in 1882, the SPR was the first organization to conduct scholarly research into human experiences that challenge contemporary scientific models.

The Spiritualist National Union (www.snu.org.uk)
The UK's largest spiritualist charitable organization was set up to unify and support the 350 spiritualist churches nationwide. Find churches in your area on the website.

The Windbridge Research Center (www.windbridge.org)
The Windbridge Institute is an independent research organization consisting of a community of scientists with varied backgrounds, specialties and interests, specializing in Consciousness Studies, After-Death Communication and mediumship.

University of Northampton, UK (www.northhampton.ac.uk)
Research group studying parapsychology, after death communication and mediumship. (Psychology Dept: Dr Callum E Cooper)

Bereavement support

Bereavement Advice Centre (www.bereavementadvice.org)
Free UK helpline and web-based information service provided by Simplify, which gives practical information and advice on the many issues that face us after someone dies.

Cruse Bereavement Care (www.cruseorg.uk)
National charity that exists to promote the well-being of bereaved people and to help anyone suffering a bereavement to understand their grief and cope with their loss. Offers confidential counselling and support, and advice about practical matters.

GriefLine Australia (https://griefline.org.au)
GriefShare (www.griefshare.org)

US-based online support group and advice centre.

My Grief Angels (www.mygriefangels.org)
Comprehensive list of links to resources and groups to help cope with the grieving process. The resources are organised by type of loss and there is a section on international resources by country.

Scientific research

Beischel, J, and Schwartz, G, "Anomalous information reception by research mediums demonstrated using a novel triple-blind protocol", *Explore,* 2007 3(1), 23–27, https://pubmed.ncbi.nlm.nih.gov/17234565/

Beischel, J, et al "Anomalous information reception by research mediums under blinded conditions II: Replication and extension", *Explore,* 11(2), 136–142, https://pubmed.ncbi.nlm.nih.gov/25666383/

Beischel, J, et al, "The possible effects on bereavement of assisted after-death communication during readings with psychic mediums: a continuing bonds perspective", *Omega,* 70(2), 169–194, https://pubmed.ncbi.nlm.nih.gov/25628023/

Beischel, J, *Investigating Mediums: A Windbridge Institute Collection* (Blurb, 2015)

Delorme, A, et al. "Electrocortical activity associated with subjective communication with the deceased", *Frontiers in Psychology,* 2013 Nov 4, 834, www.researchgate.net/publication/259208199_Electrocortical_activity_associated_with_subjective_communication_with_the_deceased

Frisén, J, Stem cell research, www.frisenlab.org/research/

Kelly, EE, and Kelly EW, *Irreducible Mind: Toward a Psychology for the 21st Century* (Rowman and Littlefield Publishers, 2009)

Kelly, EW and Arcangel, D, "An investigation of mediums who claim to give information about deceased persons", *J Nerv Ment Dis,* 2011 Jan 199(1), 1117, https://med.virginia.edu/perceptual-studies/wp-content/uploads/sites/360/2016/12/KEL13JNMD-2011-Mediumship-Paper.pdf

Kobayashi, M, Kikuchi, D, Okamura, H, "Imaging of Ultraweak Spontaneous Photon Emission from Human Body Displaying Diurnal Rhythm", *PLoS One*, 2009 Jul 16(4), https://pubmed.ncbi.nlm.nih.gov/19606225/

McCraty, R, "The Energetic Heart: Bioelectromagnetic Communication Within and Between People", *Clinical Applications of Bioelectromagnetic Medicine*, 2004, 541–562, www.heartmath.org/research/research-library/energetics/energetic-heart-bioelectromagnetic-communication-within-and-between-people/

Muller, A, "What Is Quantum Entanglement? A physicist explains the science of Enstein's 'spooky action at a distance'", *The Conversation,* 7 Oct 2022, https://phys.org/news/2022-10-quantum-entanglement-physicist-science-einstein.html

Parnia, S, et al, "Awareness during resuscitation – a prospective study," *Resuscitation,* Dec 2014 85:12, 1799–1805, https://pubmed.ncbi.nlm.nih.gov/25301715/

Vaish, A, Grossmann, T, and Woodward, A, "Not all emotions are created equal: The negativity bias in social-emotional development", *Psycho Bull,* 2008 May 134(3), 383–403, https://pubmed.ncbi.nlm.nih.gov/18444702/

Van Lommel, P, "Near-Death Experience, Consciousness, and the Brain. A new concept about the continuity of our consciousness based on recent scientific research on near-death experience in survivors of cardiac arrest", *World Futures,* 2006 62, 134–152, www.tandfonline.com/doi/abs/10.1080/02604020500412808

Van Lommel, P, "Nonlocal Consciousness: A concept based on scientific research on near-death experiences during cardiac arrest", *Journal of Consciousness Studies,* 2013 20, 7–48, www.ingentaconnect.com/content/imp/jcs/2013/00000020/f0020001/art00001

Van Lommel, P, *Consciousness Beyond Life: The Science of the Near-Death Experience* (HarperOne, 2010)

Reincarnation and pre-birth memory research

Leveridge, B, "The mysterious girl he saw", *Guideposts*, https://guideposts.org/angels-and-miracles/miracles/gods-grace/the-mysterious-girl-he-saw/

Poonam Sharma, BA, Tucker, JB, "Cases of the Reincarnation Type with Memories from the Intermission Between Lives", University of Virginia, https://med.virginia.edu/perceptual-studies/wp-content/uploads/sites/360/2015/11/Intermission-memories-JNDS.pdf

Rivas, T, Carman, EM, Carman, NJ, Dirven, A, "Paranormal Aspects of Pre-Existence Memories in Young Children", University of North Texas Libraries, Winter 2015, https://digital.library.unt.edu/ark:/67531/metadc948119/m2/1/high_res_d/34-2%205.%20Rivas%20cx%202018.pdf

Tucker, JB, "The Case of James Leininger: An American Case of the Reincarnation Type", *Explore*, 2016 Jun 12:3, 200–207, www.sciencedirect.com/science/article/abs/pii/S1550830716000331

Further reading on spirituality

Dass, R, *Be Here Now* (Crown Publications, 1971)

Dyer, W, *The Power of Awakening* (Hay House, 2020)

Freke, T, and Gandy, P, *The Hermetica: The Lost Wisdom of the Pharaohs* (Tarcher, 2022)

Gnostic Gospels (translated and interpreted by Alan Jacobs and Rev. Dr. Vrej Nersessian) (Watkins Publishing, 2016)

St John of the Cross, *Dark Night of the Soul* (Dover Publications Inc, 2003)

Tao Te Ching (translated by Stephen Addiss) (Hackett Publishing, 1993)

The Bhagavad Gita (Penguin, 2008)

Three Initiates, *The Kybalion* (Perennial Press, 2018)

Watts, A, *The Way of Zen* (Rider, 2021)

Further reading on science and spirituality

Alexander, E, *Proof of Heaven: A Neurosurgeon's Journey into the Afterlife* (Simon and Schuster, 2012)

Clegg, B, *The God Effect: Quantum Entanglement, Science's Strangest Phenomenon* (St Martin's Press, 2009)

Esch, T and Stefano, GB, "The neurobiology of love", *Neuro Endocrinol Lett*, 2005 26:3, 175, https://pubmed.ncbi.nlm.nih.gov/15990719/

Fenwick and Fenwick, *The Truth in the Light, An Investigation of Over 300 Near-Death Experiences* (White Crow Books, 2012)

Kubler-Ross, E, *On Life After Death* (Celestial Arts, 2008)

Leininger, A and Leininger, B, *Soul Survivor: The Reincarnation of World War II Fighter Pilot* (Hay House, 2017)

Monroe, R A, *Journeys Out Of The Body* (Bantam Doubleday Dell Publishing Group, 1998)

Moody, R, *Life after Life: The best-selling original investigation which revealed Near-Death Experiences* (Harper, 2015)

Newberg, A, *How Enlightenment Changes the Brain* (Avery, 2016)

Parnia, S, *What Happens When You Die?* (Hay House, 2007)

Penrose, R, *Cycles of Time: An Extraordinary New View of the Universe* (Bodley Head, 2010)

Radin, D, *The Conscious Universe: The Scientific Truth of Psychic Phenomena* (HarperOne, 2009)

Sutter, P, "What is Quantum Entanglement?" LiveScience.com, 2021, www.livescience.com/what-is-quantum-entanglement.html

Tart, C, *The End of Materialism: How Evidence of the Paranormal Is Bringing Science and Spirit Together* (New Harbinger, 2009)

Tennov, D, *Love and Limerence: The Experience Of Being In Love*, 2nd Edition (Scarborough House, 1998)

Tesla, N, *My Inventions: The autobiography of Nikola Tesla* (Merchant Books, 2019)

Tucker, J B, *Life Before Life* (Piatkus, 2009)

Tucker, J B, *Return to Life: Extraordinary Cases of Children Who Remember Past Lives* (St Martin's Press, 2013)

Further reading on soul connections

Hart, N R, *Twin Flame Love: Soulmate Poetry* (Monday Creek Publishing, 2022)

Newton, M, *Journey of Souls: Case Studies of Life Between Lives* (Llewellyn Publications, 2010)

Plato, *Symposium* (translated by B Jowett) (Lector House, Public Domain)

Prophet, E C, *Soul Mates and Twin Flames: The Spiritual Dimension of Love and Relationships* (Summit University Press, 2017)

Rumi: The Book of Love Poems of Ecstasy and Longing (translated and commentary by C Barks et al) (HarperOne, 2005)

Weiss, B, *Only Love Is Real: A Story Of Soulmates Reunited* (Piatkus, 1997)

Further reading on mediumship and spirit communication

Beischel, J, *Among Mediums: A Scientist's Quest for Answers* (Windbridge Institute, 2013)

Borgia, A, *Life in the World Unseen* (CreativeSpace Independent Publishing, 2015)

Broad, C, *What The Dead Are Dying To Teach Us: Lessons From The Afterlife* (Watkins Books, 2019)

Cheung, T, and Broad, C, *Answers From Heaven: Incredible True Stories of Heavenly Encounters and the Afterlife* (Piatkus, 2017)

Conan Doyle, A, *History of Spiritualism* (Echo Library, 2006)

Findley, A, *On The Edge of The Etheric* (Book Tree, 2010)

Greaves, H, *Testimony of Light* (Rider, 2004)

Roman and Packer, *Opening To Channel: How To Connect With Your Guide* (H J Kramer, 1987)

Smith, G, *Developing Mediumship* (Hay House, 2009)

Steiner, R, *Concerning the Astral World and Devachan* (Steiner Books, 2018)

Williamson, L, *Contacting the Spirit World* (Piatkus, 2010)

Further reading on living with grief

Kessler, D, and Kubler-Ross, E, *On Grief and Grieving, Finding the Meaning of Grief Through the Five Stages of Loss* (Simon & Schuster, 2005)

Kubler-Ross, E, *On Death and Dying, What the Dying Have to Teach Doctors, Nurses, Clergy and Their Own Families* (Scribner Book Company, 2014)

Acknowledgements

There are so many people to thank, not least the wider public for choosing to read this book. I am full of gratitude because I know just how much those in the spirit world want to reach you with their message of unconditional love.

Thanks too to my wonderful clients, students, social media community, close friends, SAS group and closed circle members, who have openly shared and trusted me with their true stories and raw emotions. Your input has been invaluable as you have shown me there is an appetite and a need for this teaching.

To my husband, Martin, for his ever present support while I sacrificed time together to write, and to my Soul Family, with whom I continue to learn, grow and evolve, including of course, my two beautiful daughters ... pure love radiates to you beyond words.

But, extra special heartfelt thanks must go to the few who actively played a role in helping me create this book: my publisher, Jo Lal, who is quite simply brilliant, and my copy editor, Kate Latham, who just gets my vision every time. You are absolutely golden! My incredibly fantastic mum, Ann South, who goes above and beyond the call of duty and deserves more praise than I could ever articulate.

And last, but most certainly not least, to Gyles Whitnall, who has been so integral to the process of my understanding. This book couldn't have been written without him. You, wonderful soul, are heaven sent!

About the Author

Claire Broad is a medium, spiritual teacher and bestselling author. She gave her first message from the spirit world to a relative at the age of four and began developing her ability as a medium from the age of 21. She currently has over 25 years of professional experience working as a spiritual practitioner, bringing greater soul awareness and comfort to thousands of people across the world.

She is accredited as a registered and approved medium with the Institute of Spiritualist Mediums, and works with her spirit team in various ways including one-to-one private sessions, public speaking, teaching and writing. Claire is author of the bestselling books, *Answers From Heaven – Incredible True Stories of Heavenly Encounters and the Afterlife*, *What The Dead Are Dying To Teach Us – Lessons From The Afterlife* and *Heaven Sent – Soul Lessons From the Afterlife*. She trains at the world-renowned College of Psychic Studies in London, as well as running her own successful and ever growing training programme, covering areas including spiritual awareness and enlightenment, mediumship and spirit communication, soul connections and soul healing.

Claire has appeared in the mainstream media, featuring in the UK National Press and guesting on radio stations and popular podcasts such as BBC Radio 5 Live, BBC Radio 4, Howard Hughes' The Unexplained.tv and Jim Harold's Paranormal Podcast.

In 2020, Claire joined forces with highly gifted energy practitioner, Gyles Whitnall. Together with their joint spirit team, they specialize in spirit guide channelled soul healing sessions, healing for spiritual crisis and spirit release, and healing through soul connections.

How to contact Claire

To find out more about Claire's work with the spirit world or about the work she does as a team with Gyles, visit her website www.clairebroad.com. Claire would also love for you to join her over at her YouTube Channel Together with Spirit, or sign up to the mailing list on her website. You can also discover Claire on various evolving social media platforms (up-to-date details on her website) or alternatively, get in touch via Welbeck Publishing.